SHOUTING AT THE SKY

ABOUT THE AUTHOR

Gary Ferguson has written for a wide variety of national publications – including *Vanity Fair*, the *Los Angeles Times*, and *Outside Magazine* – and is the author of sixteen books on nature and science. His recent title ***Decade of the Wolf*** (Lyons Press) was chosen as the Montana Book of the Year. ***Hawks Rest: A Season in the Remote Heart of Yellowstone*** *(National Geographic Adventure Press)*, was the first nonfiction work in history to win both the Pacific Northwest Booksellers Award and the Mountains and Plains Booksellers Award for Nonfiction. ***The Great Divide*** (W.W. Norton) was an Audubon Magazine Editor's Choice selection. Ferguson was the 2002 Seigle Scholar at Washington University, St. Louis, as well as the 2007 William Kittredge Distinguished Writer at the University of Montana.

Gary is a regular presenter on nature and ecology issues for conservation-minded groups across the nation. Visit him on the web at www.wildwords.net

2009 Sweetgrass Books Paperback Edition

*SHOUTING AT THE SKY: TROUBLED TEENS
AND THE PROMISE OF THE WILD.*
Copyright © 2009 by Gary Ferguson. All rights
reserved. Printed in the United States of America.
No part of this book may be used or reproduced
in any manner whatsoever without written permission
except in the case of brief quotations embodied in
critical articles or reviews. For information, go to
www.wildwords.net

Originally published in hardcover in the United
States by Thomas Dunne Books, an imprint of
St. Martin's Press in 1999.

Cover photographs by Zach Hessler
www.naturesgiftphotography.com

ISBN 10: 1-59152-061-4
ISBN 13: 978-1-59152-061-0

FOR ERIC

CONTENTS

ACKNOWLEDGMENTS

My sincere thanks to the amazing collection of field staff and therapists who provide the sometimes startling, always incredible experience known as the Aspen Achievement Academy.

And to program managers Tony Milward, Dave Gahtan, and Rich Adams; administrative staff Mark Hobbins, Susie Duffy, and Casey Smart.

Also my gratitude to John Hendee and Keith Russell of the University of Idaho Wilderness Research Center; Marilyn Riley of Wilderness Transitions, Inc.; and librarian Bob Moran of Red Lodge, Montana. At Thomas Dunne Books, a special thanks to Pete Wolverton. Heartfelt thanks as well to my inspired assistant, Anita Anderson, for her tireless efforts on behalf of this paperback edition.

Last but far from least, my thanks and best wishes always to the kids. It was you who taught me the power of truth and worth of community – you who showed me the depth of spirit that can lie waiting in a wounded heart.

PREFACE

This is the story of a spring and early summer spent in the wilds of southern Utah with some of the most troubled, extraordinary kids I've ever met. They'd come to that desolate place—most of them very much against their will—to be a part of an exceptionally good and particularly decent therapeutic wilderness program, the Aspen Achievement Academy.

I struggled for a good half year trying to decide whether to mention this program by name. This is, after all, less a tale about the marvels of any single program (there are others out there equally as good) than it is about the power and possibility in a bunch of hard-pressed teenagers living close to the ground in a quiet patch of outback, held in the arms of a community of caring, slightly offbeat people, many of whom themselves have struggled mightily to tell their own truths, to unearth the promise of their own hard roads. Furthermore, this program, for all its good, seems incredibly fragile. Higher demand might well tempt those in charge to grow it too fast, speed up the line as if this were a business of widgets instead of relationships, send the whole thing crashing to the ground.

My decision came after a conversation with the father of a bright, hungry sixteen-year-old. Immediately following what he calls his son's "wonderful success" at Aspen came another experience, this one at a place so full of mindless discipline that within a month of enrollment his son withdrew completely and closed himself off from the world, losing altogether whatever fire had first been sparked in that southern Utah desert. "People need to know that not every program out there is doing things right," he told me. "It seems only fair to celebrate one that is."

For purposes of confidentiality, names and other minor biographical details in this story have been changed; in a few cases, composites have been created further to hide identities. Finally, to protect the privacy of program operations, the names of many backcountry locations have been altered.

FOREWORD

On a cold, bright day in the spring of 1998, I loaded a backpack, kissed my wife and petted the cats, climbed in the car and headed south to the wilds of southern Utah, there to chronicle one of the nation's most compassionate, successful outdoor therapy programs for at-risk teens. Far from hospitals or mental health complexes, miles from suicide wards or drug rehab facilities or even the well-worn couch of the psychiatrist, here the healing arose from a maze of windswept canyons, from atop tall mountains dappled with aspen and pine. The kids themselves - fourteen to seventeen year-olds, mostly from middle to upper middle class families - were smart, highly creative, and greatly troubled. Some were angry and full of fight, while others were sad, barely able to carry the weight of their trampled hearts. They were alcoholics and drug users and cutters, drop-outs and runaways. And with few exceptions, they were veterans of nearly every kind of therapy imaginable. Taken together they formed a small, yet by no means unusual sampling of our nation's struggling youth. As one sixteen year-girl told me, sitting under a juniper tree in the Red Desert, "We're just the ones who got caught."

All these years later, it's still hard times for American teens. Abuse of prescription drugs is at an all-time high - part of a teen addiction problem that's grown in America at a rate twice that of other developed countries. Conduct disorders and a wide range of other so-called behavioral problems continue to mushroom. The National Resource Council recently predicted that one out of every four kids aged ten to eighteen are now at risk of being incapable of living productive adult lives. Even those not currently struggling with acute problems face challenges unknown to earlier generations. Recent studies suggest that by the time he reaches age seventy-six, today's fourteen year old will have spent a staggering twenty-eight years exposed to various kinds of electronic stimuli. From an evolutionary standpoint, humans have never been subjected to the overwhelming noise being tossed at today's teenagers. One seven-year investigation, led by Dr. Brian Primack of the University of Pittsburg School of Medicine, suggests that teens who experience five-and-a-half hours of radio, television, internet and computer games per day – an amount actually below the current average – will by age twenty-one be at significantly greater risk of developing depression. Some neurologists worry such exposure to computers and video games may actually be altering the wiring of the brain; one effect may be a retarding of development in the brain's frontal lobes, which influences everything from the development of social skills, to impulsive behaviors.

*   *   *   *

Given that nature has proven a powerful setting for healing across thousands of years, it stands to reason that, at the very least, it could provide teens with the chance for much-needed respite in these hectic times. Yet in truth, it's doing much more than that. When it comes to treating modern teen drug addictions, for example, Dr. Keith Russell of Western Washington University has shown that compassionate outdoor therapy (as opposed to so-called boot camps), is enjoying success rates significantly higher than traditional treatment programs. Meanwhile, research released in 2009 by Dr. Salli Lewis of the Center for Research, Assessment and Treatment Efficacy, showed participants in wilderness therapy enjoyed significant, lasting improvement in solving problems related to attention-deficit hyperactivity, conduct disorders, aggressive behavior, depression, and suicide.

Science has much to say about why such positive change occurs in nature. But it's also worth hearing a few insights from the young people I actually followed through the wilds of southern Utah. Last spring I was able to reconnect with nine of the twelve participants you'll be reading about in this book; happily, all but two are leading challenging, fulfilled lives: A pediatric nurse. A social worker. A custom tile artist. A drilling rig forewoman. A professor. A teacher. A therapist. (Of the other two, both young men, one continues to wrestle with alcohol, while the other – years after a severe brain injury - ran afoul with the law for petty theft.)

"It was the first place where what I did mattered," said Susan, who arrived at Aspen struggling with depression. Like others, she was alluding to the fact that being comfortable in nature requires not only physical exertion (for her, this proved especially helpful), but also a high level of personal responsibility and thoughtfulness toward the group. Sit on the side of the trail for three hours and pout if you must. Staff will ask what's wrong and try their best to engage you. Yet in the end no one will force you to move. When the group finally does get going, though, arriving late to camp, frustrated by having to cook and set up their shelters in the dark, it's going to dawn on you how your choices affect everyone. Natural settings teach, wrote John Burroughs, far more than they preach. Unlike the strange fantasy worlds portrayed on television, in programs like Survivor, the reality of being in the wilds is that the group is never stronger than its weakest member.

"It was the first time I've ever known beauty," said Nancy, echoing a comment many made immediately following the program. In every culture, on every continent, natural beauty has been a primary resource for helping people through difficult times. It wasn't that people thought it a panacea. Rather, beauty was used to gain fresh perspective on the world - an essential nudge toward the kind of clarity that often eludes people in times of emotional pain.

In the heart of the Middle Ages, when much of Europe was being urbanized for the first time, leaders of the Catholic Church found themselves with a vexing problem. The faithful were sinking into a kind of malaise, a low-level depression of spirit known as "acedia." Desperate to solve the problem, the fathers put future saint Thomas Aquinas on the case, certain that his devotion, not to mention his brilliant powers of deduction, would shine light on the problem. The trouble, Aquinas would later explain, was quite simple: people were suffering from acedia because they'd somehow lost their ability to be in touch with the beauty of the natural world around them. If these kids are to be believed, beauty is no less powerful today than it was then.

"It was the first time I've known what I think," Sarah told me at the end of a two day solo. Again, the chance for deep quiet, for a space in which to become familiar with the thoughts, dreams and "self talk" that occupy our waking hours, is for most young people next to impossible. Perhaps it's no surprise that the harried, dispirited lives of so many – struggling in what educator G. Stanley Hall described long ago as a "hothouse culture, where everything ripens before its time" – would be soothed in the fluttering aspen forests atop Thousand Lake Mountain, under dark skies full of stars.

One might imagine that our current disconnect with nature could be easily repaired. Yet today's compassion-based wilderness therapy movement has become a race of sorts - a struggle to stay one step ahead of an increasingly common view that says nature, at least outside its use for sport or entertainment, is just too harsh of a setting for therapy. Our growing discomfort with wilderness, along with tragic stories about a handful of fly-by-night outdoor programs, has left some seeing nature less a gift, than a punishment. Actually, today's best accredited wilderness programs are remarkably safe, with injury rates lower than their institutional counterparts. Yet no matter how compassionate and well regulated the program, no matter the sterling credentials of the staff and therapists, subjecting children to seven weeks in the outdoors, with occasional chilly nights and hot days, with the chance of bugs and wind and rain, is for some people hugely disturbing. We're mistaking comfort, for kindness.

Shortly after the initial release of *Shouting at the Sky* I was a guest on a popular national call-in radio show. In the course of the hour-long conversation two women from different parts of the country phoned to share their experience with different wilderness therapy programs. One woman's son was enrolled at fifteen in an urgent attempt to break his cocaine habit; the the other woman's boy, sixteen, had been living on the streets of Philadelphia, running with a gang. Without that wilderness intervention, each one said, their boys would likely be dead.

"Still," sighed the host, "isn't it a shame we've come to the point where we have to throw our children to the wolves?"

In the face of such fear, we might do well to consider an old Ojibwa story called *Butterflies Teach Children to Walk,* which reminds us that the young of all creatures grow not by having everything done for them, but rather by striving, by reaching for what they want. I recently spoke with a young man I first came to know in Utah – at the time a tough, angry boy from the Midwest, who in the end would need six years to finally get sober and turn his life around. Yet it was his time in the wilds, he insists, that provided him with the first critical step on his long journey. On hearing that some people consider such therapeutic programs abusive, he was incensed. "It wasn't abuse," he told me. "It was hard work. And nobody wants to work that hard any more."

Compassionate wilderness therapy is not a fix for broken kids. How well teens do in the months and years following their experience depends a great deal on what they go back to at the end of the trail. Furthermore, many times a young person will "fall off the wagon" several months after getting out of such a program, only to later become rooted in healthy living. Yet as many of the students you're about to meet continue to remind me, wilderness therapy is a lot more than a time out for bad behavior, or an experience whose relevance quickly fades in the rear view mirror. The skills and perspectives gained in these wind-scoured canyons, in the shade of these quiet forests, to this day remain for them critical tools in their struggle to live well in the world. Perhaps biologist Rachel Carson was right: those who contemplate the beauty of the earth, she said, create reserves of strength to last their entire lives.

In twenty-five years of writing projects, I have never found a gathering of people – students, field staff and therapists alike – more committed to kindling thoughtful, intentional lives. During a recent personal tragedy of my own, when my dear wife of twenty-five years was killed in a canoeing accident, in my darkest days, heartbroken and hopeless, I often found myself thinking of that time a decade ago, in southern Utah, on the trail with those extraordinary kids. What they were struggling to learn, I've come to understand, is what we all have to learn in the wake of a shattered life: How to make room for the pain. How to open our eyes, put our faces to the ground, and begin gathering up the shards of our calling. And ultimately, with a little help from those around us, to refashion life into something whole again - something beautiful enough to color the deepest blemish, something hopeful enough to bind the most terrible wound.

Gary Ferguson

April, 2009

EVERY CHILD SHOULD KNOW SOME SCRAP
OF UNINTERRUPTED SKY, TO SHOUT AGAINST. . . .

—Edna Casler Joll

AUTOBIOGRAPHY
Frank, Age Sixteen

My father is an Episcopalian who has been divorced too many times to count and drinks too much.

My mother goes to church every Sunday in hopes that somebody will notice her there and think she is a good soul.

I never admired my father in his Jaguar with his pretty wives; I admired a homeless man who would let the ashes fall into his lap.

I spent my schooldays being kicked out of Catholic schools and my nights sleeping on the beach waking up with a hangover.

I've spent too many days in the library on speed.

I've lain down on sacred land.

I've seen beauty.

I've had visions.

I've spent summer days on a park bench with Buddha.

I've come up short in the city without a dime.

I've admired stories and fallen in love whenever I drink.

I've traveled and always found my way back home.

I am sorry something caught my eye but I didn't turn to look.

I've had conversations at a thousand miles per hour for days non-stop.

I've felt spirits and seen energy.

I have a bad back from sleeping in the bathtub.

My life is pressed like a flower between these pages.

I cannot sleep.

I am anticipating a revolution.

But still, I can't find myself.

CHAPTER ONE

COYOTE GIRLS

THE MIDDLE OF Utah's Red Desert, two, maybe three in the morning. Light from a full moon is spilling all over the place— down the shoulders of Caineville Reef, across the long, flat sweeps of sage and rabbit brush and greasewood, through a thin braid of dry, nameless washes, onto the faces of seven teenage girls scattered across the ground at the edge of a box canyon, hoping for sleep. Lisa and Jenna are having weird dreams again, twitching and mumbling, setting off on what seem to be conversations, passing off a slur of words and grunts, even instructions: "Not that way," Jenna is saying. "Go left. It's over there." I'm trying to remember it all, give the words back to them in the morning on the off chance they might hold some kind of meaning.

A few feet away Nancy is poking Tricia in the ribs, trying to get her to stop snoring. And beyond that, under the only tree within a half mile, is the new girl, Brenda, the one who just went on suicide watch. Such a strange routine for her now: the drawstring taken from the hood of her sleeping bag, the laces pulled from her boots—just in case. A blue tarp spread tight across her bag with two staff lying on the outside edges, one on either side of her, the better to feel every move she makes.

If this were your first week in the field, you'd probably be thinking it'd been one hell of a day. Carla had her first try at leading the group on a night hike, laying open a personality that was something like a cross between Joan Crawford and an aerobics instructor. No one took it well. And then that thing with Brenda. Around midnight she decides to sit in the middle of the road, refuses to walk any more, starts cursing, spitting on us. Says what would really make her happy is if all of us would burn in hell. Before it's over she manages to raise everyone's hackles, even stalwart Jenna and the normally tranquil Nancy, sending them over to staff with teeth and fists clenched, asking if they could "hit her just once. C'mon, just once!" Not surprisingly, when we got to camp, sometime around one in the morning, Lisa called a group to talk about it. But instead of telling Brenda what a bitch she was—and that would have been pure Lisa— she said only that she understood Brenda's loneliness, that she knew about the anger she felt at being here. That things would get better. That if she needed to talk . . .

So much craziness, and on one of the most beautiful nights I've ever seen. The kind of desert night that feels like a gift. Delicate. The air filled with the smell of juniper and sage, desert holly and cliff rose, sandstone and alkali dust. And out beyond camp hundreds of sego lilies, one to a stem, their ivory blooms glowing in the wash of the moon. Lying awake through these wee hours I'm thinking maybe all this wouldn't be so hard to get my head around—wouldn't seem so filled with contradiction—if my culture hadn't spent the last hundred years thinking of the wilderness mostly as some kind of tonic: sedative, blood-pressure medicine, speed. The wilds as the place we go to smell the pine and the rain, dangle by ropes from the chins of mountains. It's been such a long time since deserts and woodlands were places of confrontation, stages on which to wrestle with shadows and cry for visions, holy lands hiding strengths that go unsuspected in more common hours.

The old people of this place, the Paiute, knew full well that beauty and craziness would be found together like this, standing hand in hand. Paiute creation myth tells how long ago the earth was danced by two brothers, Coyote and Wolf. Wolf with his perfect, wholesome vision of the world, a creator who never wanted anything more than an abundant life for the people, a life free of anguish, free even of death. And the younger Coyote, spoiled, mischievous, the glib talker who time and again pulled his older brother away from those plans for perfection. And how after a time Wolf went away, leaving the world to unfold according to the imaginations of Coyote. We cast our fate with Coyote, said the Paiute. And so our lives are driven by this strange mix of urge and shadow, by schemes going out into the world meaning to be clever, coming back full of pain.

Now these smudged, sweat-stained girls, kids who never knew of or cared a damn about the Paiute's brother gods, lying here in the shadows of these same ancient canyons, wrestling with Coyote things of their own. With their habits of crack and

speed and crystal meth. With late-night trips to the police sta-
tions, to the streets, to the suicide wards. Early in the afternoon
with girlfriends at school, in the toilets, throwing up lunch.
Hammering together pieces of whatever's in reach, trying to
survive. Like Nancy a couple of days ago, walking down that
dusty trail, talking about her bulimia: "How could I deal with
things if I didn't throw up?" she said. "What else is there in my
life I can control?" Then later, around the fire, before bed, she
starts rapping on the bottom of one of the tin cans we use to
cook in, and then someone else starts in with her thumbs against
the bottom of her blue metal cup, and then three more cups
and a pair of wooden spoons, until there's this heady thrum
drifting out across the desert—in some moments disjointed, but
in others, perfect. And right in the middle of it a coyote comes
up to the edge of the bench that runs along our camp to the
south, gives three bright barks, turns, and walks away. All of us
sitting there looking at one another, amazed; never slowing the
rhythm, though, never stopping that drumming.

"That coyote," Nancy says over breakfast the next morning, as if only then was it proper to speak of it. "It was awesome." And she slipped that memory into her pocket, and she's
been walking with it ever since, all across this empty desert,
drinking from it like a spring, smiling over it when the weight
of her pack and the long black nights start pressing on her shoulders.

Fifteen hundred miles to the northeast, in a well-trimmed suburb
on the outskirts of Chicago, the day is beginning in the most
god-awful way. Five o'clock in the morning, and two big, thirty-
something strangers are standing at the head of Ray Macias's

bed, one with a muscled hand on his shoulder, rocking him out of a tequila sleep barely three hours old. "Ray," the guy is saying, louder now, but still calm, no hint of anxiety. "Ray, it's time to get up. We've got a busy day ahead of us. Let's go. Get up and get dressed." The man turns on the lamp next to the bed. Ray scrunches his eyes, lays his arm across his face.

"Who the fuck are you? Whaddaya want?"

Now the other guy is turning on more lights, opening the curtains, pulling back the covers. "My name's Lee," he says, pausing to squat beside the bed. "And this is Dave. It's a big day for you, Ray. A new start. Everything's gonna be all right, but we have to go now."

By now Ray's awake enough to wonder where his parents are. Then he hears his mother down the hall, sobbing. And the muffled voice of his father.

"Your folks love you, Ray. They're sending you someplace where you can get it together again. Your stuff's all packed— it's right here by the door. We need to get going. C'mon, get up now."

Now Ray is yelling for his parents; then *at* them, shrieking, cursing; and when he finally breaks to catch his breath he notices they're moving not toward his room but down the stairs. His mother is calling out in this desperate-sounding voice, thick and broken, "I love you, Ray! I love you!" And then the real shock: His father, the guy with no emotion, Mr. Stoneheart, is out there bawling like a little boy. Ray will tell me later that it was then that he felt the fear breaking loose, the sour taste rising in his throat, this feeling like it was the end of the world.

By five-thirty Ray is being ushered out the door. His body is hunched over and he's jerking away from Lee's hand, refusing even to look at his parents, who are standing in the kitchen doorway looking very much like children themselves, trembling, clutching at one another. Lee and his partner give them an understanding look, tell them again that everything will be all right, that they'll call the minute they land in Salt Lake. The door closes. The car starts. The men and the boy drive away.

Ripping Raymond Macias from his old life in Chicago and sending him off to live in the wilderness for sixty days, Jack and Marie will say later, was absolutely the last resort. Three weeks after Ray leaves for Utah, they'll sit shoulder to shoulder on a white couch in a living room splashed with framed prints of various Latino artists, holding hands. Looking tired. Looking guilty. Saying how this is the final stop on a long, painful road lined with twelve-step programs and therapy and group counseling, psychiatric hospitals and visits by pastors, and wave after wave of "tough love."

"We heard about wilderness therapy from a psychiatrist," Marie says. "That's the latest psychiatrist, Doctor Briles. We've been through a few. He told us he's seen it happen—kids who didn't respond to conventional treatment getting better out there. No guarantees, of course." It's probably because of comments from her sister, the raised eyebrows of her neighbor, but Marie seems eager to point out that this isn't some sort of boot camp, that it's a kind program, built on therapy. She lets go of her husband's fingers for a minute, leans forward, rests upturned fists on the knees of her jeans. "I don't know if you can possibly understand how drained we are. Not just Jack and me, but Ray's younger brothers, too. How hopeless we feel." She pauses for a few seconds, lost in thought. "Think of what it would be like to have someone you love suffer a terrible stroke—bad enough you couldn't reach them anymore, couldn't communicate at all. The relationship just evaporates. Now add to that kind of pain a sense of—I don't know what else to call it—menace. Like when Ray and two of his friends decided to rip off a Quik-Mart a few blocks from school. Or when Jack found a revolver wrapped in an old rag, wedged into a corner shelf of the workroom. When I found out he was selling crack out of his bedroom. We feel like victims. Like hostages."

"At least out there he'll be safe," says Jack, who sounds skeptical about his son's chances of success. "If nothing else the outdoors will give him that. I know it's just two months. But Ray hasn't been safe for a long time." What he doesn't say, what surely must be no less appealing, is that he and the rest of his family will be safe as well.

Marie says part of the deal with this program is that she and Jack had to agree to go to therapy too, at least once a week, for the entire two months that Ray's in Utah.

"I don't have a problem with that," Jack says. "These past few years have done terrible things to me. I've been beaten down. My guard is up all the time. It's a habit now, the way I survive. That isn't what Ray needs to come home to if he wants to make a fresh start. Then again, I've gotta tell you, at this point I don't have much energy left for new beginnings."

Ray, of course, has little choice but to begin again. Three weeks from now, while his parents are sitting in the living room wringing their hands over having sent him here, he'll be smack in the middle between the life that was and the life to be. No one knows whether anything will come of his experience. But by then Ray will tell me that, for the first time in years, at least there's the feeling of not having to fight. In the days ahead he'll walk through these windblown valleys with a bandanna tied around his head and on his neck a piece of sinew strung with brown dry juniper seeds. He'll make fires by spinning wooden spindles against sage fireboards until embers form, and cook in blackened cans set on coals at the edge of the flames. He'll write poems and tell his story. Before it's all over he'll walk this desert south to north and back again. He'll climb mountains. He'll wake up in the hollow of the night under a sky shot full of stars. And while to the few people who'll spot him and the other boys from behind the windshields of their Suburbans and Explorers all this may look like the stuff of summer camp, from where he stands, it will seem like nothing less than the flowering of a tribe.

CHAPTER TWO

CLAN OF THE CRISES JUGGLERS

IT'S NOT THE geology or the biology lessons, or even how to make a bow-drill fire. Not the stern cautions to keep hold of the bag full of medications, complete with the tale of a kid who figured out how to hide Ritalin in the back of his throat and cough it up later when no one was around, trading it to other kids for hot chocolate. Not talk around the fire about the risk of burnout—"an overload of unbelievable drama," as one of our trainers, a woman named Paula, calls it—or how days off had better be filled with plenty of singing and dancing and good books if we're to have a ghost of a chance of staying sane. Not the constant reminders that we aren't here to cure or to heal— merely to try to give kids an experience they can use, whenever

and however they want. Not the importance of keeping war
stories out of Wanda's drive-in and the Aquarius Cafe, where the
ears of all Wayne County—"Wayne's World," as some like to
call it—will forever be upon us, how you don't really have to
do anything strange in these parts to be considered a freak.
Nothing so significant as that. The memory that always comes
first when I think back on eight days of training is the embar-
rassment of spending the first forty-eight hours having to count
out loud whenever I head off the trail to take a leak, announcing
my whereabouts, just like the kids have to, so those in charge
can keep track of me.

It begins in the middle of a windswept, glorious desert
nowhere, at the second or third tick of a spring that will prove
as beautiful as anyone has seen in a long time. The cottonwood
leaves are just beginning to pop, a million of them lining every
wash, driven by the miracle mash that produces a green so
bright and unblemished and full of electricity that no matter
how many times I see it it looks impossible, dreamed up, like
that weird, unripe-lime-green crayon that Crayola came up with
in the 1960s, which all year long seemed good for nothing until
the first blush of spring, when suddenly it made perfect sense.
The lupine leaves are out, the cow vetch is starting to blossom.
The desert holly is covered head to toe with tight little fists of
blooms, every one of them wearing the color of the sun and
smelling like good perfume.

Eight newcomers, hoping to become field staff in an eight-
week wilderness therapy program for "at-risk" teens. At risk of
what, exactly, depends on who you talk to. In the best cases,
at risk of driving their parents absolutely nuts; in the worst—
and in truth, the worst is far more common—at risk of self-

destructing. Only one kid out of a hundred actually comes here because he or she wants to. Most already have plenty of interventions under their belt—therapy schemes, rehab centers, detention, boarding schools—you name it. And then one day some therapist throws up her hands, tells Mom and Dad it's time to try something really different: It's time to try the wilderness.

And so this group of wannabe instructors, men and women mostly in their twenties from as far away as Florida and Vermont, talented and passionate and eager to feel they're doing something worthwhile, few with any clear sense of just what they're getting into, none with any guarantee of a job. There's Elizabeth, tanned and strong, fresh off a two-thousand-mile hike up the Appalachian Trail and five months living in Tibet. And Beth, quiet, timid. Emily, who plays guitar and sings with a voice like sweet clover, and Laura—vulnerable, determined, full of intuitions.

There's Kate, too. Good-hearted Kate, daughter of a New York City actor who in his mid-thirties chucked it all to go back to work the family apple orchard in central Vermont. Kate grew up there, dancing and singing among the Jamaicans who came every year to work the harvest. As an artist she has a fondness for weaving works out of natural materials, and from the look of a few photos she passes around during training, she's remarkably good at it. My favorite is a shot of an antique lace wedding dress brocaded with thousands of seeds and burrs and then hung out among the trees near the orchard. It looks like the gown some Celtic spirit bride would wear, rising on spring nights to plead with the trees to put forth apples. Like most of Kate's art, this one will be picked at by the winds, tattered by rain and snow, fall apart, come to rest in pieces on the ground.

Among the guys is Florida Dave—so attentive, honest, and

sincere that you'd hand over your kids, your dog, and your life
savings to him and never think twice about it. Dave headed west
out of Florida five months ago, spending most of his precious
dollars on gas for a two-thousand-mile sojourn across the country to join a woman who turned out to be less than thrilled to
see him. Dave's a longtime vegetarian, and when the only job
he could find to make his share of the rent was as a waiter in a
Sizzler—well, he took it as a sign, or at least as the last straw—
figured that maybe this love affair wasn't meant to be after all.
He tells me that the whole relationship was exactly like a piece
of verse he read in the training guide for this program. "Here,"
he says, thumbing through his already dog-eared copy of the
manual, pointing out a little ditty called "Autobiography in Five
Short Chapters."

CHAPTER ONE

I walk down the street.
There is a deep hole in the sidewalk.
I fall in.
I am lost . . . I am helpless.
It isn't my fault!
It takes forever to find a way out.

CHAPTER TWO

I walk down the same street.
There is a deep hole in the sidewalk.
I pretend I don't see it.
I fall in . . . again.
I can't believe I am in the same place!
But, it isn't my fault.
It still takes a long time to get out.

CHAPTER THREE

I walk down the same street.
There is a deep hole in the sidewalk.

I see it there.

I STILL fall in ... it's a habit.

My eyes are open ... I know where I am.

It's my fault.

I get out immediately.

CHAPTER   FOUR

I walk down the same street.

There is a deep hole in the sidewalk.

I walk around it.

CHAPTER   FIVE

I walk down another street.

In the end Dave floated his ex-partner a tearful farewell, climbed into his pickup and headed west to California, where he spent some time working in a meditation retreat, heard about this program from a friend, and decided to give it a try. Yet another example of how not just the kids, but a lot of those who end up working with them, seem to be standing at their own crossroads.

There's also Park City Dave, a wisecracking Alaska fisherman who's rubbed elbows with death on forty-foot seas, and Todd, a big, muscled snowboard instructor from Park City who believes that, no matter what's ailing you, a bout of good, hard play is one of the best tonics around. And Mike, who calls himself a recovering addict and recovering research chemist, who's looking for something more. He's the closest thing to a hippie we've got, having rolled into the little Mormon town of Loa in his faded white '76 Chevy van, with big flowers and the name "Lulu" (from a Grateful Dead song) painted in big red letters on the side.

And still one more Dave, this one from Grand Junction,

Colorado, thirty-seven, done with the stress of trying to run his own business making outdoor clothing, looking to build a life helping kids, maybe one day starting a program in which entire families can jump into the wilderness and work on their stuff—group therapy at its best: in the dirt, on the mountain, at the river. Grand Junction Dave is the gadget man, in love with all those compact, clever little devices you see in outdoor catalogs—things like folding skillets and collapsing cups and sawed-off toothbrushes.

In all, there's a fantastic sense of quirk and ramble to these young lives. A willingness to live out of cars and sprawl in sleeping bags in the living rooms of friends—an almost giddy courage to roam the four corners of the globe and walk among people whose language they don't understand; on any given day, grateful for the chance of something unexpected. Indeed, what most distinguishes them is their willingness to put themselves out of their comfort zone. Break the frame. Not that they don't limp a little now and then, get out of bed some days and trip over old baggage: alcoholic mothers, abusive fathers and uncles. Addictions. Being overweight as a kid. Depression so weighty it's pushed some to the brink of suicide. "To do this work it helps if you're a little crazy yourself," one veteran instructor told me the day I arrived in Loa. "It helps to know about pain. It helps to know the value of the struggle."

At forty, there's no missing the fact that I'm very much the old man of the bunch. One more outsider who drove into Loa in an old Chevy van—officially as a writer, looking at wilderness as a setting for what might be best called a rite of passage—unofficially because something just plain pulled me here. There's a weird familiarity about the whole idea of troubled kids ending up in the wilds. Maybe it's no more than the fact that

America has such a long history of pushing its outcasts into the sticks—hookers and drunks and opium hounds to the gold-mines, brawlers and ruffians to army outposts on the frontier, thieves and petty crooks to the timber camps. More likely, though, it has to do with the fact that after all this time, I can no longer imagine being broken without a wild place to fall apart in.

We've come to this work at the tail end of a strange, tur-bulent few years. In the spring of 1994, a sixteen-year-old boy named Aaron Bacon fell in with a poor excuse for a wilderness program, also in Utah, called North Star. He was weeks into it when he started complaining of severe stomach pains. The staff didn't take him seriously. He ended up dying. Wilderness ther-apy in general has been equated with that tragic, senseless death ever since. Several good programs, including this one, either folded in the wake of the catastrophe or nearly did. When I told friends about spending several months here, more than a few figured it was some kind of investigative trip—that I was going undercover to catch people whipping kids with bulrushes or something. One education consultant I talked with warned me not to get carried away by what I saw here—that this was a good program, but that good programs are the exception, not the rule.

Bacon's death definitely brought important questions to bear on an industry in which, given the remote location of the work, those inclined to run shoddy programs can and do so. On the other hand several instructors I've met who were once stu-dents here themselves have a somewhat different take. Without the intervention of a sound, compassion-based program like this one, they say—a final door opening after every other kind of therapy had failed—they would've been dead long ago. More than a few recent graduates, as well as their parents, say the same thing. "You can hate what happened to Aaron Bacon," as one father from Denver put it, "without needing to hate the whole idea of a kid going to the wilds to heal."

Trainees met for the first time a couple of days ago, in Loa—got the nuts and bolts of how things work, were introduced to instructors and therapists, nurses and directors and educators. This morning we went on a field trip of sorts, learning about the geology and biology of the place, which is probably a good thing, given that field staff is responsible not only for helping Johnny cultivate a vision of life beyond crack and crystal meth but schooling him for credit along the way. It was at the end of this field trip, after hours of Tony, the field director, helping us get a handle on the fact that Navajo sandstone is stacked on top of the Kayenta formation—which is stacked on top of Wingate sandstone, which rests on top of the Chinle formation and the Moenkopi—that we got dropped off out here in the desert with our water and our packs, rendezvousing with our three trainers, Paula, Rich, and Dave.

There's enough anticipation in the air to set the lizards twitching. Trainer Dave kicks things off by collecting everyone's watches, bracelets, necklaces, and rings, as well as any stray food we may have in our pockets or packs, putting it in plastic bags and handing it to Tony. Florida Dave has half a bag of sunflower seeds left, which he's kind enough to pass around, sensing, as the rest of us do, that there isn't going to be a whole lot in the way of snack food for some time to come.

It's the first step of a plan to start our backcountry education by treating us pretty much like the kids we'll be working with in the weeks to come. While Dave collects jewelry and food, Paula tells us to unload our wonderful double-stitched internal-frame Dana and Osprey and Gregory packs we're so fond of and load them into the back of the pickup, at which point Tony offers us his good wishes, climbs into the truck, and rumbles back up the dirt road for home. Each of us has a big blue tarp to lay out our belongings on, which in turn gets tucked and folded into something like an egg roll. We tie it off with parachute cord, attach straps made out of seat belt webbing, and hang it from our shoulders. Fully loaded we look like a cross between bohemians and vagrants, models for the L. L. Bean April Fool's catalog.

We'll begin, Paula tells us, as mice. That entry-level creature slot, low as you can go, beneath coyote, buffalo, and eagle, in which kids spend their first forty-eight hours in the wilderness. To be a mouse means to be on separates, slightly apart from the group, no talking to other students. Eating something like peaches and water and granola—fare that some say helps cleanse the system of whatever drugs may still be running around. Were we students we'd also be asked to come up with a few written lines about why we think we're here, along with what it is we can offer the group, which as trainees we more or less do anyway, but verbally, sitting in a circle in the sand. No "future information" is given to any student, unless he or she is an eagle, so questions about how far we're going, when the next break is, what's on tap for tomorrow, go unanswered. And then that thing I mentioned earlier: asking permission whenever we have to relieve ourselves and then having to count out loud while we're doing it, lest we suddenly give in to the urge to make like wolves and run for home. If we prefer, Paula tells us, it's okay to sing instead of count, though personally I find it hard to come up with a song appropriate to urinate by. The first time I'm out here peeing behind a rock I end up count-

ing to ten, over and over again, thinking how mundane that
would get if it went on for long, like if I were out here squatting
for fifteen or twenty minutes with a bad case of constipation.
To make matters worse Dave yells after me, says he can't hear
me, that I need to turn up the volume.

It's hardly a breakthrough notion to divide a program like
this into levels—mouse, coyote, buffalo, eagle—each requiring
knowledge of a long list of specific hard and soft skills, each
holding out more freedom and responsibility. While back on the
home front such platforms might seem trite, out here a lot of
kids reach for them with surprising eagerness, are perfectly willing to embrace the rituals and ceremonies used to mark them.
Even more surprising is how many of these mostly city-bred kids
get way into the animals whose names they wear. Maybe they're
just bored. Then again, could be they take to the fact that animals in general are simply out there doing their thing—none of
them, to the great relief of the kids, with the slightest concern
about what sort of meaning a teenager might care to invest them
with.

Besides, we're not talking about some thoughtless drift up
the food chain. You'd be hard-pressed to choose a better poster
critter for the first full round of struggle a kid faces here in the
wilds than coyote—the survivalist, a canine that knows better
than most how to adapt in the face of adversity. Kids are asked
to be coyote-like by showing a willingness to try new things:
put themselves out there in a group, learn the kinds of skills
that make for a manageable life in the wild.

Next up the ladder is the buffalo, a massive herd of which
lives right next door to us, in the toes of the Henry Mountains.
Buffalo are communal animals, acting in ways that ensure the
survival of the group. Out in human land, of course, this is a

quality we love to tout as one of the great cornerstones of adulthood. Kids at buffalo level are expected not only to support others trying to deal with their stuff but to find ways of getting their own feelings of anger and fear and issues of relationship out in ways that don't unravel the rest of the group.

And finally the eagle, which—despite us having dragged its feathers through the mud for decades as the mascot for everything from credit cards to insurance companies—in these parts is meant to spark something more than notions of security and consumption. Around here staff is likely to point out the eagle's habit of rising higher in the face of oncoming storms—getting above the danger, using that broader perspective to figure out what to do next. Ironically there's an old Native American proverb about eagles, one that few people around here have ever heard, one that could have been plucked right out of the lives these kids left behind: "If an eagle seeks the praise of a swine," the saying goes, "it will have to spend a lot of time wallowing in the mire."

We start hiking about an hour before dark, and by the time we stop for our first break the sky is full-on black with a slice of grapefruit-colored moon. I'm liking it. And from the looks on all the other faces, I'm pretty sure they're liking it, too. Of course that we can be so happy about our lot in life out here in the big open points to some major differences between our little outing and that of the kids. None of us had an ex-linebacker walk into our room at five o'clock in the morning with a duffel bag of clothes, nudge us awake, and tell us to get dressed because we were headed for Utah. None of us had parents so afraid we'd run away, maybe even turn violent, that they lured us to Utah with a cock-and-bull story about a ski vacation in Park City, only to pass us off to escorts at the Salt Lake City Airport. True, a lot of kids know they're coming here, but even then it's usually a choice between this place and something they consider even worse. All in all the kinds of setups guaranteed to blind you to the sweet, bleak beauty of a night like this, the way the rims and the mesas are going soft in the moonlight, the feeling that life has come down to the smell of sage and the sound of our own footsteps splashing through the creeks and scraping against the sandstone, the croak of frogs along Sweetwater Creek.

These kids you'll be with, an instructor named Mike told me, are like all kids. They're looking for some measure of power, some kind of control over their lives. Aren't we all? I think as we walk on through nameless arroyos, past clumps of grease-wood and juniper, on and on through the night. Let's face it, if Paula and Dave and Rich were arrogant about the power they have over us tonight, which they never are, I'd bet that more than a few of us would be as tempted as any kid to flip them off and make for home.

Around midnight we call it quits, seven, maybe eight miles up the trail. A good walk but hardly an expedition. Actually our trek is just a miniversion of a time not so long ago when there was no such thing as a mouse, when all the kids of a group started together, going through something called impact. Impact meant walking long and hard, twice as far as this, maybe more—not as some kind of punishment but as a means of pushing buttons, of getting the kids to define their stuff by acting out, with the side benefit that they'd go until they were way too tired to piss and moan anymore. The old-timers here say that impact had the effect of solidifying the group, of building bonds that lasted the entire program. "With impact it was intense right from the start," says a senior field instructor named Ben. "We didn't wait for a month to find out what was going on—the kids would tell us in the first day or two."

In the end, though, the whole idea of mass starts troubled the people holding the purse strings, who balked at the fact that the company was paying for kids to be in holding situations until enough students were on-site to begin a group. Impact went the way of the dinosaur, launching the era of staggered admissions— the era of the mouse. Not that the shift was all bad. At least now the newcomers have a chance to watch and learn from kids who've been in the program awhile—the leaders, the buffalo and eagles. And naturally, what other kids say and do out here can carry a lot more weight than anything the staff might offer.

By midmorning of the next day we're off mouse, alternating the last of the hike to training camp with serious sit-downs in the dirt, talking about the proper responses to all kinds of issues we'll need to be aware of in the weeks to come. Already some of us are shedding some cherished notions we had about what was going to happen here. Huddled under a tree to escape the heat of the noon sun, Paula tells us she'd guess that more than 50 percent of the kids who come here end up going on to other programs, usually therapeutic boarding schools; Dave and Rich place the number closer to 60 percent, especially in the winter months, when the kids who come here tend to be a bit more hard-core. This is an intervention, they tell us.

It's not that we can't see the need for that sort of thing, for the going on to someplace else, especially if the family is on a loose footing. For that matter the whole idea of nuclear families being somehow sacred would two hundred years ago have been heresy; back then, and for centuries before then, the faithful were far more concerned about spiritual families than ones made of flesh and blood. What's so troubling about the idea of teenagers passing out of one rehab door and then another, from this therapeutic boarding school to that one, is a lack of sustained community of any kind, flesh and blood or otherwise. Oh, we'll get used to it. But for the moment it leaves some of us thinking that the only village raising the children in this neck of the world is a loosely woven tribe of crisis jugglers. And then only if you can afford them.

As trainees we haven't been here long enough, aren't smart enough to know that we'll go crazy if we take on the full weight of such unfairness. Mike, the recovering research chemist, is still talking about it late at night, in his sleeping bag, trying to unwind. He says he's glad to be able to lie here and look up at the stars, hear the distant yip of a coyote, because for the moment that seems like the only shred of evidence there's any sanity left in the world.

"Beyond the procedures," Dave told us, "there's only this: Do your job with love. Give these kids every bit of positive energy you can muster. At the least you'll go a long way in keeping a bad situation from getting worse." I think about that a lot in the minutes before sleep. And I can't quite convince myself it's enough.

The next morning is golden, full of hope, my first inkling of the kind of emotional roller coaster that goes on for anyone who does this kind of work. The good comes in large part thanks to the arrival of the program's education director, Lavoy Tolbert. In the coming weeks I'll hear sixty-three-year-old Lavoy referred to by staff as wizard, shaman, and magician. More amazing is that the kids will be every bit as much in awe of him, though they'll use slightly different language to show their respect, referring to him as either "the bomb," "the man," or "the pimp." To say that Lavoy is into spending time out-of-doors is like saying that the pope is into going to church. While in the early 1970s the rest of America was packing up station wagons and heading to some state park or the KOA, Lavoy was grabbing a knife, a little cordage, maybe a tarp, walking with his children into the wilds to spend a few days fending for themselves. "Few people actually ever see Lavoy coming," Dave tells me. "He just sort of walks out of the trees or the scrub and suddenly he's there"— a fact that does nothing to diminish the magic. Lavoy is a fierce champion of the wilderness part of this program. He fairly bristles at any rumors of changes that could water down the power of a kid simply being in this wild place. Therapy is good, Lavoy will tell you. Curriculum is good. But, as Outward Bound founder Kurt Hahn liked to say, when you come right down to it, the mountains can speak for themselves.

Lavoy teaches like nobody I've ever seen. It's not just a matter of knowledge, though he's way down the highway on that. It's more this uncanny knack he has of talking with you for five minutes and from that brief exchange seeming to know exactly the questions to ask to allow you to find solutions on your own, in your own style of learning. Doesn't matter if you're depressed, distracted, have ADD (attention deficit disorder), are angry. Kind of a Socrates meets Kreskin sort of thing. An hour after meeting Lavoy I find myself flashing on my entire school career, wondering what life would have been like if my classes had been led by men and women like this. "When I was teaching," Lavoy tells me, referring to his twenty-seven years spent in the public schools, "I used to stand at the front of the room and look at those thirty students and think 'there could be the next Einstein.' And that tickled me! Tickled me like bubbles rising in seltzer."

Lavoy is of modest build, even slight, but taut like cable. His right arm is halfway bent, held close to his side, the hand half open. At fourteen Lavoy was out on horseback, doing a little cowboying on the family ranch, ended up lassoing a calf that had been munching on locoweed, was a little crazy. It charged. As the calf ran by the flank of his horse the rope got wrapped around Lavoy's arm, halfway up, jerking him out of his saddle and dragging him across the ground, slicing through the skin down to the bone, severing the nerves so badly that his arm and hand never functioned again. He's perfectly willing to talk about it, answer any questions. It is, after all, no small part of who he is.

Lavoy has come out of the woodwork today to help us with astronomy, one of some three dozen lessons included in the program's curriculum. With Lavoy, though, we don't just sit in the dirt and listen. Hardly. Ten minutes into it he has us standing in a big circle sculpting all kinds of astronomical phenomena by using our bodies as the planets, as the sun and the moon and the stars. Fifteen minutes into it we've become this great circle of people spinning and rotating out in the Utah desert, Lavoy tossing questions, his eyes lighting up at every "aha!" look he spots flashing across our faces. Before it's over, some two hours later, the most subtle, confusing notions of constellation movement and the spin of the seasons and eclipses are rooted in our heads—for some of us, the first time ever, understanding pouring into our brains as easy as rainwater into a kettle hole. After he leaves, walking off into the wild to who knows where, Florida Dave comes up to me, shaking his head. "Lavoy's the man," he says, and all I can do is nod my head and stare up the wash, into a cluster of junipers where I swear I saw him just a second ago.

After Lavoy it seems a bit of a letdown to start stuffing our heads with procedures again, most having to do with keeping the kids safe, along with some good, if somewhat astounding, stories from the field. Mostly we talk about using natural, or logical consequences, instead of punishments; about how this program has to do with influence, not control. There are definitely discipline-based, military-style programs out there—more of them all the time. This isn't one of them.

Dave makes the case for why, at least with the kinds of kids in this program, there isn't any need to rule with an iron fist. One of the beauties of being out in nature, he says, is that kids get the chance to see a direct connection between their behavior and their experience. You can't manipulate the wind or the rain or the mountain, or talk your way out of the coming of darkness. There's no Mom and Dad to feel sorry and rescue you, no one to go live with who might be more inclined to let you off the hook.

"A kid will sit down on the trail, refuse to move, so we'll stop the whole group and wait. We tell him what we'd like to see happen, but we don't enroll ourselves in his drama. Either he'll do it or he won't—it's really okay either way. And at some point—maybe it's fifteen minutes, maybe it's three hours—he'll give us a wide-eyed look, finally know that we mean it. And that's a revelation. Kids say, 'Wow, my mom tells me stuff like that all the time and then bails me out twenty minutes later. You're more hardheaded than I am.' "

It's a favorite pastime among trainees in the off hours to

talk about discipline-based programs—specifically, how coarse
and disagreeable they seem. "It seems strange," Grand Junction
Dave offers, "to try to mold kids with heavy doses of discipline,
then expect them to go back into a world where that sort of
outside influence is completely absent." It's an interesting point,
especially considering that most psychologists use as a measure
of maturity the shift from a so-called external locus of control—
reacting to outside influences—to an internal locus of control,
which means making decisions in your own behalf. Still, Aspen's
therapeutic director speculates that for perhaps 10 to 15 percent of the problem kids out there, control might be the better
way to go. "It's probably most appropriate for kids on both
extremes of the behavior scale. Older, more hardened kids
who've successfully used anger and control for years to get what
they want. And then the flip side—kids who are total victims,
the ones who won't take care of themselves at all." She says it's
definitely possible to run a good program based on discipline,
but that you have to be very careful, because such an approach
is linked to power, and power can be easily abused.

At the moment I have my own bias against such an approach, though I confess it's not based on any real experience.
Just a knee-jerk reaction to the director of a large discipline-
based program in the Southwest telling one of his field staff that
the secret to success is to "beat the shit out of the kids until
they fly straight."

It's late in the afternoon when we turn to the matter of making
fire. Being in the generation of outdoor ramblers drilled in the
need to use backpacking stoves, few of us have given much
thought to fire as a daily piece of living in the wilderness. It's

not that we're ignorant of the appeal of campfire—most of us know full well that flames can coax things out of people that might otherwise never find voice. But the fact that the only fires ever started out here are by bow and drill, and that every student has to master the technique in order to eat hot food, at this point seems little more than one of those clever camp tricks meant to pad a kid's pockets. I'm happy enough to learn it. But then I'd be just as happy to learn how to juggle, or make a birdcall, or do a backflip.

The mechanics are fairly simple. Find a piece of sage heartwood or cottonwood root and chop it down to a board maybe two inches by eight inches by a half-inch thick. Next, carve a spindle—if you have a cottonwood board use cottonwood, if you have sage, use sage—round as you can make it, perhaps an inch thick and eight inches long. Then a bow, roughly the size and shape of a violin bow, strung with cord or a shoestring, or, if you're really into it, with cordage made from natural fibers. And finally a socket rock, which is a palm-size flat stone with a natural indentation you grind out with another harder rock, like chert; lacking such a stone, an anklebone from a cow or a deer skeleton you find lying in a wash will do fine. Wrap the spindle in the bowstring, laying one end in the depression you've carved into the fireboard and the other into the socket rock, kneel down, with the wrist of the hand holding the socket rock locked against your shin, begin bowing like a cellist until you see smoke, increase the pace for ten seconds. Stop, knock the punk into your nest of bark or grass, and hold the nest face level and blow and blow, and by God there will be flame. At least that's what they tell us.

What none of us counted on was how much building a bow-drill fire makes you want to focus, to solve the problem like some great tinkerer, as if you were Thomas Edison or something, even if on most days that just doesn't seem your nature. Is the spindle too big or too pointed, the bowstring too loose, the downward pressure on the socket rock too light? Is your spindle arm locked against your shin properly? Is the channel cut into the fireboard far enough below the spindle hole to collect the embers?

Obviously the payoff of hot food is a great incentive to keep after it. But the truth is, it goes beyond that. In the coming months I'll see kids with such severe ADD they can't hold a thirty-second conversation within a few weeks be perfectly willing to spend an hour focused on the bow drill. It's as if there were some kind of genie hidden in the wisps of smoke rising from the fireboard, showing them parts of themselves they never imagined existed—patient, untiring, clever parts. Clearly, along the way will be fits of rage, kids throwing their bows into the woods or busting them across their knees, stomping on their nests. But always, sooner or later, a deep breath and another try. In a sense making fire isn't so much about accomplishment as empowerment. A big fat favor granted by the wilds. The key to heat, food, and warmth, and in that the best bounty of all— a ground floor to what the day before was fear without bottom. Somehow it seems only right that so many of the world's cultures would weave myths celebrating these glowing embers as gifts, that they'd come to know the twirling of spindles as mother giving fire.

The field part of training ends with that great staple of every wilderness rite of passage for years beyond counting—the solo. Alone in the desert, on a sweet spring night when you can smell the holly without even trying, when the old junipers are flying their bark like prayer flags in the evening wind. While the kids typically go out for at least two nights, we'll be gone only one. Each of us has a bag of lentils and rice and a potato, some oats, a sleeping bag and bow-drill set, and sealed away in a Ziploc bag, a story about the great Shawnee leader Tecumseh. Stories are used a lot around here, and not in the old quaint way of summer camp. A folklorist I know in Tennessee says that in a lot of cultures if young people did something wrong they weren't admonished for it. They weren't beaten or grounded or sent off to live with relatives. They went to the storyteller. The storyteller would sit down with them face-to-face, gather his breath, and slowly, carefully begin unraveling this tale or that, something filled with intrigue, rich with holes and doorways into which a kid could slip his need like a key and claim part of that story as his own. It's hard to say why programs like this lean so hard on Native American stories. Maybe in order to cast young heroes as struggling for courage, nobility, and have it come even close to being believable, you have to plant them in a strange and distant culture, one where the adults seem bound to the same ideals.

I find a spot about a mile from camp in a green glade thirty feet by twenty, surrounded by enormous, gnarled junipers. I set up my tarp, gather wood and juniper bark for nesting, bury my potato in the dirt, make my first solo fire on top of it—nurse it, close my eyes and inhale the smell of it, then fill my metal cup with water and lentils and rice, and set it at the edge of the flames. Dinner under way, I settle in with the Tecumseh story, a tale from when the future leader was a young boy, maybe eight. Late in the fall Tecumseh is told by his father that he's to begin a great trial, one step on his way to manhood, to obtain his *pawawka*—a kind of amulet that warriors would wear, gathering strength from it throughout their lives. Because a *pawawka* is so powerful, his father tells him, it will not come easy. Nothing of importance comes easy.

Each morning at dawn Tecumseh must gather his intention, walk down to the riverbank, and then jump into the cold water. Day after day, week after week, on through four moons, well past the time when the river grows bitter cold and choked with ice. The only thing that will keep him from freezing, he's told, is the fire burning inside. At first there are others there watching, lending support, but in time they drift away, leaving Tecumseh to tend his ritual all by himself. And that, of course, is the hardest time of all. But he stays with it, and on the last day he breaks the ice, jumps in, and grabs his *pawawka* from the river bottom—a beautiful rock, unlike anything the people have ever seen. A touchstone to his inner strength.

Something tells me that the waking up in this desert every morning is the jumping in the river: the *pawawka*. As far as that goes, the water already seems plenty cold enough to make even the trainees shudder, what with the six days of stories we've gathered about runaways and suicide watches, about digging kids out of the snow at dawn and trying to convince them to walk when all they really want to do is lie down and pull winter over their heads and go to sleep for good. About the girl who came last week who can't seem to muster the will to go on, the one with the boyfriend who shot himself to death in the front seat of his car with her sitting there beside him.

"These are young kids," Paula told us. "Just getting them to identify an emotion, to share, is a huge accomplishment. Believe in the program, the place. That's what's going to push the issues to the surface." Still, let's face it, for most of us our first reaction on seeing a drowning person is to jump in and try to save her. It's going to take a certain restraint to row the boat into deep water, to within shouting distance, and offer what amounts to swimming lessons.

We come off solo the next morning in silence, just as we left, find a great meal waiting for us, courtesy of Paula and Dave. Afterward we circle up and talk out the experience. Grand Junction Dave in particular is nearly beside himself with revelations, talking on about how his solo left him wanting to swear off his high-tech habit, saying he realized that his folding aluminum trowel and his gadget knives were just another layer of stuff between him and the wilderness. A way to feel less afraid. "There's another part of it too," he says. "All that stuff—some of it's very expensive stuff—seems weird in a place that has nothing to do with money. Out here it doesn't matter whether you're rich or poor—everyone faces the same dangers. You can be president of the United States or some guy living in the gutter, and you can die of thirst just the same, can lay down your bag in a gully and get swept away in a flash flood."

Around noon the trainees are told to pack up and be ready to head off for their first overnight with an actual group; I'll be staying behind with Dave and Paula. After several years working here, this is Paula's last week, and she's in a reflective, melancholy mood. At one point it's just her and me in camp, and we sit in the shade of a big juniper, watching ants and fiddling with sticks and absentmindedly drawing in the sand. She plucks a piece of pitch off the ground, rolls it between her fingers, tells me if I grind it up it'll make great kindling for my fires.

Unlike some of the staff, Paula doesn't share the hard road of having been abused, of getting in trouble with the law, of wrestling drug monkeys. In fact she's pretty clean—bright, ar-

ticulate, passionate, a woman destined to end up in charge of
things. She says what led her here was her strong love for nature—that even as a kid she could see the power of it. "When
I was little, whenever I was upset I wanted to be outside. If I
was really sick, like I had the flu or something, I'd drag myself
outdoors and lie under the apple tree. I'm a good listener, a
good facilitator. Part of the reason is because of all the time I
spent in nature. I learned patience there. I learned to be quiet."

I ask her about the kids she's been working with in this
program. Are they really not far removed from a lot of young
people out there today? She thinks it's true. "Look," she says,
leaning forward, wrapping a pair of dusty arms around her
knees. "It takes a lot of time to make the money you need to
have the standard of living society seems to expect. Parents are
incredibly busy trying to make the incomes to give their kids
certain things. But the one thing they aren't giving them is time.
We talk a lot with these kids about where they get the things
they learn, their perspectives. You know what they say? They
say they learn from television, and they learn from their friends.

"You're going to hear this a lot: 'My parents couldn't take
the time to deal with me so they sent me here.' You'll see a lot
of cynicism in these kids, and part of it's based on the fact that
they've learned coping skills like the ones we teach, yet no one
seems able to take the trouble to help them put that stuff into
their lives." She offers as example a sixteen-year-old boy who
came in last week, furious at having been sent here. "They leave
me home for years," he told the staff. "I've been doing drugs
all along, right from the beginning. Now all of a sudden my dad
finds out about it and he wants to do something. Why didn't he
pay more attention in the first place?"

Paula says a lot of the kids who come here have attention

deficit disorders, but that they also have low self-esteem, and that's the problem that gets them into so much trouble. "Why? Because people haven't told them they're okay, haven't taught them how they can get along in other ways. They're one of thirty-five or forty kids in a classroom, led by a teacher who's been trained to teach to the kids who learn the same way most other people do. Out here ADD kids learn. They learn a lot." Paula makes the point that there's an explosion of alternative programs right now—dozens of them, springing up all over the country, fueled by a growing population of kids who don't have anywhere else to turn, for whom nothing is working.

Dave comes back from running shuttle late in the afternoon, asks if I'd be willing to help out with a little experiment. The plan is for me to take an article of clothing—I choose an old pair of Levi's—and run off into the desert, dragging the pants behind me through the sage and the cactus to see if Annie the bloodhound can sniff me out. Annie is the latest program volunteer, lending her nose to the search efforts that are launched whenever one of the kids decides to blow the wilderness and run for home. Tony, the field director, is Annie's trainer; he'll be on the other end of the leash, encouraging her, patting her on the head for staying on task. In truth I get a little overenthusiastic, end up running down washes and over rock banks, through the piñon groves for well over a mile before snapping out of it and concluding that enough is enough. I realize I may have pushed the envelope when I hear Tony, a big, stout man, panting from nearly a hundred yards away. I peer out from my hiding place behind an enormous juniper to see Annie literally dragging him through the wash, like in the Westerns, when they'd tie some poor sap to the back of a horse and run him around the *despoblado*.

Annie finds me, all right, slobbers like a leaky hose all over my lap, vacuums up a couple of handfuls of cheese, and calls it a day.

"Keeping the kids safe," Tony pants. "That's our first concern. If they run, no one's gonna find them faster than Annie." Soon it will be running season, he says, referring to the warm days and mild nights that make getting out—or at least attempting it—seem like a far more reasonable alternative. I stare across the landscape—nothing, not a shred of civilization in nearly four hundred square miles—trying to decide whether running is more an act of desperation or of courage.

And just like that the training trip is over. We pile into the trucks, Kate and me and a new therapist, Brett, in the back of Florida Dave's Mazda pickup, under the shell, sweltering in the heat, sucking dust and passing water bottles, heading for Loa. Unlike another new therapist here this week, Jason, who after two days has managed to remain disturbingly neat and clean, Brett has lost some of his preppy look under a coat of grime. He wears a dirty baseball cap, backwards, stray tufts of blond hair poking out along the sides; it's a youthful look, a cross between a twelve-year-old kid standing in the outfield and a Mormon rapper. His new boots are coated with dust. It's the look he needs to wear when he's working with the kids—something that says I'm out here in the trenches with you. A look that goes way past being another clean-shaven shrink in a sports coat, watching the clock, billing by the hour.

The truck is rattling on the washboard road like a can of stove bolts on a paint mixer. Yet we talk the whole way, philosophizing in shouts about whether a good program is better than a not-so-good family. About how tough it is in the days of gangs and drugs to follow the wisdom of ancient myth that says you have to get lost in order to find yourself—defy the people of the village, if you will—without losing yourself for good. How for most of human history the evolution from child to adult has been fueled by scary, uncertain, humbling days in an uncluttered place, crying for a new way. How America's rituals seem to be lying in shambles, our adolescent rites of passage reduced to pay-to-play programs like this one, used not to empower kids as a matter of course but merely to pull back the ones who are standing on the brink, hopeless, all but lost.

Five miles down the road we pass one of the all-girls groups pushing two-wheeled carts loaded with packs and a cast-iron Dutch oven and big blue barrels filled with water. One of the girls passes near the window of the camper shell, a tall redhead maybe sixteen, staring in at us. She's incredibly strong looking, tanned, greasy hair tied back with a bandanna and a face full of dust, wearing a grin that seems part proud, part defiant. It's Jenna, I'll learn later—a sixteen-year-old wannabe gang-banger from Portland who was hanging with an older guy who liked to hit her. "Her parents sent her here to get fixed," one of her friends will tell me. "Right now they're back home sitting in their living room, hoping she's going to come back all nice and everything. But look at her. She's so strong. She'll confess to her own crap. But she'll also call her parents on theirs." My God, I'll think, imagining the day her parents come to get her. What a reunion!

For some reason seeing Jenna reminds me of something Lavoy said the other day, when he magically appeared out of nowhere to teach us astronomy. He'd just finished telling me about his arm getting damaged in that roping calamity when he was a kid. "Do I wish things were different?" he said of the accident, which was exactly what I was wondering. "Not really." And then he flashed this disarming grin, the kind of look that sometimes passes between old friends when one knows that he's about to say something already understood by the other, something the both of them found out a long time ago. "After all," he said, "who would any of us be without our pain?"

CHAPTER THREE
THINKING LIKE A MOUSE

I DON'T KNOW what I expected the escorts for this place to look like. Something at least close to those former pro football players some parents use to get their kids from the house to Salt Lake City, somebody big enough to blow off the curses, the threats, the occasional kick or punch. Which is why I'm a bit taken aback this morning when I meet escorts Lou and Ray in the parking lot at base—married, smiling sixty-somethings, more the kind of people who as a teenager I would've picked as my grandparents than someone plucked from the front line of the NFL. Karen is there, too, a thirty-two-year-old "raised on country" mom with a bright smile and a strong hug who picks up kids and hauls them the four hours from Salt Lake City back to

Loa with oldies tapes of classic goofy tunes like "The Monster Mash" and "Itsy-Bitsy, Teeny-Weeny, Yellow Polkadot Bikini" blasting out of the speakers of the Suburban, and, even more surprising, as often as not somehow coaxes sing-alongs out of the angry, confused teenagers sitting in the backseat.

"This is a pretty typical assignment," Karen tells me as we climb into the car. Four hours to Salt Lake to pick up three teenagers—two boys and one girl—carry them back to base for physicals, outfit them with gear, take them into the backcountry, drop them off with instructors who'll walk them into the wilds to join existing groups. Between sips of coffee from Lou and Ray's thermos, against a dawn sun flashing west to the Tushar Mountains, are stories from a hundred trips like this one, picking up not only kids bound for this program, but from the youth prison in Grand Junction, Colorado, taking them under court orders into another, more military-style program known as AYA. "We love all the kids," Lou is saying, about to shock me once again. "But the AYA kids are really special. You should see the looks on their faces when they come out of that jail, high-stepping and waving their arms, celebrating what it feels like to finally be free of handcuffs and leg shackles. The way they look up at the sky, stare out the window to the mountains. To kids in the other program this seems like terrible punishment. But when you've spent months locked up in a cell, it looks like freedom."

We stop for gas at a convenience store in Scipio. As he's paying the bill Ray reaches over to a rack of candy bars, takes one for each of the kids we're picking up, smiles self-consciously when he sees me watching, tells me how much the kids like chocolate. A minute later we're loaded and rolling again, up 120 miles of interstate, finally breaking west for the Salt Lake City

Airport. Thirty minutes out Karen opens a folder full of papers, takes a look at some rather murky-looking Xerox pictures of the kids, reviews with Lou and Ray what each is supposed to be wearing. In Keith's file—a sixteen-year-old from Indiana—is a handwritten note. "Possible runner," it says. Sometime last month, the story goes, Keith decided to bolt from boarding school wearing only his underwear. Somehow he was picked up by his friends, but they ended up dumping him back out along the highway, where the police eventually caught up with him. His father wasn't pleased. He gave Keith a choice of either coming here or spending two years at a therapeutic boarding school. We sit in the short-term parking lot going over the arrival schedules one more time, decide how we should split up— who'll get each kid—check our watches, and walk into the terminal at a fast clip.

Susan, from Witchita Falls, is the first to arrive. She's sixteen going on seventeen, wearing overalls, with straight, shoulder-length hair and plastic-frame glasses, looking very much like the smart kid on the block. And painfully timid. After our initial greeting she stands with her shoulders hunched over, unsure, as if she were protecting herself against whatever questions or other demands we must be about to lay on her. Last fall was the first time Susan tried to kill herself, taking an overdose of depression medicine, which got her a fast trip to the suicide ward. About a month ago she felt the same hopelessness all over again, but to her credit managed to let her parents in on it, telling them she needed help, saying how maybe it was time to go back to the hospital. When the hospital stay didn't seem to be doing much good, her therapist suggested something different. "When she said an outdoor program," Susan will tell me later, when the reality of where she is starts to dawn on her,

"I thought she meant some sort of summer camp."

Keith comes next. A small, wiry kid with a disarming grin—smart as a whip, asking lots of questions, listening to everything the adults say, noting the layout of things, scoping out the situation to get a better handle on his options. As we walk through the airport I notice him scanning every cranny and corridor—studying things, I'm imagining, figuring the odds of escape.

And finally Kevin, at 250 pounds, every bit as big as Keith is small. Kevin wears a purple T-shirt half in and half out, his shoes are untied, and there's a smudged, bright green golfing cap tilted on his massive head. If Keith gives the feeling that he's taking it all in, forever computing, Kevin looks as though he'd just as soon curl up in a gate chair and go to sleep. I can't decide if he's slow to get excited about anything, or just resigned to the deal the youth court cut with his father's attorney when he got busted for stealing: Come here or go to jail.

On the trip back Lou and Ray are up front, Karen and I are in the middle seat with Susan between us, and in the back are Kevin and Keith. It takes fifty miles for Keith's eyes to stop roaming—watching the interchanges, scanning the interior of the Suburban. At one point he catches my eye, points to the holes in the ceiling of the roof of the car where there used to be a pair of speakers. "What's with this?" he says. "Did some kid go crazy in this thing and rip out the stereo or something?" Kevin finds that pretty funny.

While the boys are trading nervous laughs in the backseat, Susan seems increasingly withdrawn; her willingness at the airport to exchange at least the occasional pleasantry has vanished, and now she barely answers our questions at all, more often than not shooting back a sarcastic-looking scowl, as if anyone seriously expecting her to make small talk when her world is falling apart has to be a little on the stupid side. The farther we go, the more she tends to slump in the seat and tilt her head down, until before long her hair has fallen around her face, a curtain keeping the rest of us out. Even a stop at Burger King, where Lou and Ray and Karen buy everyone a generous last round of fast food, doesn't seem to help. If the ride down is this unsettling, what will she think when she finally sets foot in the wilderness?

It takes forever to get out of Salt Lake City. Spilling down the Wasatch Front is an almost endless run of big, boxy houses and shopping islands filled with chain stores, bleeding ever southward into the old rural towns named after Mormon fathers: Lehi, Orem, and Nephi. Progress, some are calling it. When the Mormon pioneers arrived in this valley in 1847 nearly all were traditional Democrats, having followed the lead of their founder, Joseph Smith, a staunch anti-Republican who had aspirations for the presidency. But by the end of the 1800s the church was aligned with a number of large, and ultimately very successful, capitalist ventures. In time church leaders began approaching the faithful looking for "volunteer" Republicans, and that's pretty much how things have gone ever since. To this day the Wasatch Front is a bastion of Republicanism and free enterprise, home of the so-called success industry—a remarkable stewpot of day-planner companies, life-journey workshops, books, and seminars; this year the Franklin Covey Corporation alone—"supporting individuals, families, and organizations in accomplishing what matters most to them"—will have sales of over $400 million. Pundits have for decades been snickering about the statue of Brigham Young in Temple Square—his back to the church, his hand outstretched to the bank across the street.

Still, it seems oddly fitting that Kevin and Susan and Keith, and all the other troubled kids from troubled places across the United States, would come to heal among a people whose religion more than any other describes itself as pro-family, pro-kid. A religion only too happy to give millions of dollars for commercials reminding parents to spend more time with their children, husbands to take a couple of extra minutes to be with their wives. In truth, if Keith or Kevin had been from a devout Mormon family and had drifted even half as far into their crazy brand of drugs and delinquency, as likely as not right now they'd be off working at a potato co-op in southern Idaho or a cattle ranch in Wyoming, or any of a hundred other sprawling farm and livestock operations owned by the Mormon Church. Overwhelmed by the faithful. (Not that there weren't plenty of teens even in good old Deseret—the original Mormon name for this region—who gave their elders no end of grief. The leader of the Wild Bunch was a Mormon boy from Circleville by the name of George Leroy Parker, aka Butch Cassidy, and most of his gang was Mormon, too. As were the Swazey Brothers, the Ketchum Brothers, Gunplay Maxwell, and Keith Warner—Butch's mentor, and arguably one of the most accomplished outlaws of all time.)

Six weeks from now I'll be standing with Kevin in a meadow near the crown of Boulder Mountain, and he'll tell me that while he knows nothing about Mormons, he's no stranger to church. He'll talk about years spent in pews and on folding chairs at the First Assembly of God, flanked by his family, singing the songs, saying the prayers. And how, when he was around thirteen, the time his life started to unravel, it all began to seem like nonsense. "The adults do all this money-grubbing. Then they use the church to hold that up, to justify it—to make themselves feel good about the screwed up way they're living.

Why would I want to be a part of that?"

A hundred miles down the road, and Keith has lost his spark. He rubs his chin with his thumb and forefinger, looking queasy, as if his stomach is turning at the sight of these big yawns of wind-scoured valleys, at the old men in coveralls and earflap hats tottering into the front door of the Down Home Cafe in Scipio; the sad-looking woman in a gray wool coat with greasy hair, walking her mutt in a ditch puddled with ice. The friggin' end of the world. We pull into a Town Pump for gas, and Keith says he needs to use the rest room. Karen walks into the store with him, waits in a corner of the store with a clear view of the men's room door, just in case he decides to bolt. In truth, one of the reasons escorts stop at this place is because there aren't any windows in the bathrooms, which tends to make their lives a lot easier. "The urge to run," Karen tells me, "is going to get stronger the farther out of the familiar we get. You may or may not think about running when you're angry. But it's definitely an option when you're scared." At first Keith seems surprised, then pissed off to see us standing here by the potato chips watching the hallway like a couple of prison guards. He stomps out of the place, spits on the sidewalk, opens the door to the Suburban, crawls inside, slumps down in the seat, and tries to sleep.

Ever so slowly the farm fields give way to long runs of sage—and as we climb higher, to squat, gray-green huddles of piñon and juniper. What began as gentle swales along the inter-state are building into mesas, into cliffs and arroyos, the land deepening, taking breath, until by fifteen miles out of Richmond all hell has broken loose, leaving us wrapped in an upheaval of rust- and cream-colored reefs and canyons. I turn around once more to say something to Keith, try again for some kind of connection, but he's fast asleep, head tilted against the rear window. At Fremont Summit Ray checks his watch, pushes a little harder on the gas, sends us flying down the lee side of the mountain like a tumbleweed hooked to a spring wind.

Back in Loa our first stop is the clinic. Each kid gets a physical and a blood test from a remarkably calm woman doctor who asks if anything's ailing them, what their recent drug and alcohol use has been, if they have any condition that might keep them from being physical. It's nearly eight o'clock by the time we finish and head to base, where the kids get the lowdown on equipment, as well as instructions for making those curious packs out of rolled tarps and nylon seatbelt webbing. Before any of that, though, comes another sort of examination, this one done behind a closed door with a Do Not Disturb sign hung on it, a supply room filled with tarps and pants and sweaters and caps, hiking boots and canteens and Green River Knives, cordage and socks and underwear and tin cups. I stand by a stack of wool pants while Shawn asks Keith to empty his pockets and the plastic grocery sack he's carrying and place everything in a box that will be labeled, sealed with duct tape, and put on a shelf in the basement for safekeeping. The sum total of Keith's wealth comes to $9.41, a book of matches, and a nearly empty pack of cigarettes; in the bag are three giant packages of Carefree gum, more half-empty cigarette packs, a ball of hemp twine he uses to braid with, and an old library book—an adventure at sea.

Next Keith takes off every stitch of street clothes, gets a quick once-over to make sure he's not holding on to something he shouldn't be. He looks so damned vulnerable standing there—stark naked, stripped of his smokes and his trinkets, a slight, wiry little body hunched against shelves of pack frames and khaki clothes. One look at his face, and it's all I can do to not wrap him up in one of the wool blankets, toss him in my van, and make for Indiana, for his home.

Around nine o'clock I catch a ride out to the field to join an all-girls group, number 3. Susan will be coming later, so for now it's just me and a student named Carla, who actually managed to leave the wilderness for an afternoon at her therapist's request for a psychiatric evaluation. Randy, who normally manages food supply, along with his wife, Marcia, are captain and navigator of an old, faltering Dodge truck, steering us under the starlight down a tangled maze of dust-laden roads on a two-hour tour to the base of the Henry Mountains. Randy and Marcia don't have kids of their own, but they talk of the ones in this program as though they were the closest of family, confiding with me at one point how tough it is for them to let those with problem parents go back home at all. In my short time at base I've twice already heard Randy going to bat for the food, scrapping to keep nonessential goodies like extra cheese and brown sugar and canned peaches. "I don't care," he tells me. "Kids working that hard, you need to feed them."

Randy and Marcia are relatively new in the wilderness-therapy business, having taken these jobs after being forced to sell their small grocery store last November in the wake of a shiny new Foodtown coming to Loa. The place had been in the family for some twenty years. Not just a grocery store, Marcia assures me. A gathering place. A home away from home. "It feels like a death," she says. "We used to have chairs around the store for the men who had nowhere to go—the bums; things for the kids who missed the school bus and couldn't get hold

of their mothers. The salesmen used to laugh at me because
when they'd come by to take orders I had to pore through stacks
of coloring books to even find their catalogs."

Carla and I ride together in the back, in the jump seats.
She wears army pants and an olive green T-shirt, and her dark
red, curly, altogether unruly hair lies quiet for the moment under a red bandanna. Her glasses are smudged. She looks like a
bookish young woman from the 1940s, on foreign soil, heading
for the underground. After four weeks she's well tanned, and I
can't help but notice the strength of her forearm muscles. When
I ask if she worked out at home she just laughs, gives me a
"Yeah, right" kind of look, pulls back her T-shirt sleeve and
raises her arm to show me her bicep. "It's from being out here,"
she says. Carla tells me she was sent here in part because of
drugs, but mostly because of trouble with her mother. In the
course of our ride she proves to be funny, eccentric, incredibly
smart, and full of sarcasm. She's the first student with any time
under her belt I've met, and I'm eager to hear how things have
been going. "It's kind of like this," she tells me, in what through
the coming weeks will prove to be one of the most common
yet wisest remarks these kids make: "I'm here, okay? And since
there's really nothing I can do about that, I might as well make
the best of it. This thing is about being present, living one day
at a time. In the end that's your only choice."

Around eleven o'clock Randy points out the driver's window to a small two-track heading off through the sage to the lip
of a ravine. "That's where Group Three started today," he tells
me. "They're on carts, you know," referring to the five-hundred-
pound, two-wheeled wooden handcarts on which kids spend at
least a couple of weeks during their stay. It suddenly dawns on
me that this is the group we rumbled past when we were head-

ing out of the field after training. In truth, I've been thinking
about those carts ever since, remembering that the girls looked
like a handful of lost Bedouin in search of a homeland.

While this program has no church ties, handcarts are an
obvious leftover from Mormon pioneer days. In the mid-1800s
the church was doing lots of recruiting in the economically hard-
pressed regions of Cornwall and Wales—at mills and in mining
towns so ravaged by poverty that the mere thought of gaining
a little farm somewhere in America, making a fresh start, and
paving their way to heaven besides was for many impossible to
resist. Thanks to Brigham Young's Perpetual Emigration Company, getting here was incredibly easy. Using moneys donated
by wealthy Mormons around the world, hard-pressed wannabes
were given full escort across the Atlantic, guided up the inland
trails all the way to St. Louis, then outfitted with a wagon and
supplies and a team of oxen.

Immigrants were supposed to pay back the moneys spent
getting them to Utah, but for many such restitution proved difficult. As more and more people showed up at the docks in
Liverpool, eager to join the flock, the coffers of the Perpetual
Emigration Company got squeezed harder and harder. So Young
hatched a more economical plan. Mission heads in Europe were
told that those wanting to come to Utah but short on funds
would still get the guided tour all the way to St. Louis, but from
there they'd have to forgo the wagon-and-oxen part of the deal
and instead carry their supplies in wheelbarrows and handcarts.
So that's what they did. Assembled into groups of tens and fifties
and hundreds with a captain over each group, exactly as
Young's one and only revelation had instructed it be done, they
loaded up their tools and their babies and their cookpots in carts
exactly like these and pushed west out of St. Louis over more

than a thousand miles of hot, rugged prairie and mountain trail.

The fact that these same carts would end up in a program for troubled teens has nothing to do with playing pioneer, and everything to do with the fact that pushing one with three or four people—usually one or two in the front at the yoke bar, and two in the back—absolutely requires working together. I'm told that the hard feelings and bad attitudes, which on most days can easily stay hidden, will rise to a fever pitch in a single mile of pushing carts. If just one person doesn't play the game the cart will wander all over the place, and that generally makes life miserable for everyone. If the point is to dust off the hot buttons and make sure they get pushed, evoke all the responses that don't work in a kid's life in order to help him or her find ones that do, handcarts sound better than tag-team therapy with Freud and Jung. Tony tells how one day a few years ago he got an urgent radio call from one of the instructors in the AYA program, the guy panting on about how his group had just found an ax lying along the road, and now everyone was taking turns with it, chopping their cart to pieces.

Incredibly we don't reach Group 3's camp for several more miles, up a tangled, cobbly road climbing nearly fifteen hundred feet into the foothills of the Henry Mountains. I can barely conceive of six teenage girls managing such a feat, but Carla shrugs it off, gives me a look laced with pride and resignation. "What can I tell you?" she sighs. "We're an awesome group." We meet one of the instructors beside the road, well before the actual camp. "We try to keep vehicles—really, anything having to do with civilization—well away from the kids," Randy explains. "No sense breaking the feel of the wilderness any more than you have to." That one, I'm thinking, has Lavoy written all over it.

It's cold outside, the thermometer in the high twenties and still dropping. The girls have been in camp only about an hour, and the place is humming with a certain organized chaos. Lisa is sick, throwing up in the sage, and Sara, wearing the dirtiest face I have seen on anyone over the age of five, is setting two coffee cans full of water on a smoky fire she just made with her bow drill. Tarp shelters are being tied to the trees, Nancy is off digging a latrine. Jenna—the girl I saw out of the truck cab window when we were driving out of the backcountry after training, the one that looked so strong, so gnarly—is tonight's cook; I find her rummaging through the food bags, complaining loudly about the fact that they've managed to eat all their tortillas again, two days before resupply.

The staff this week includes Elizabeth, the strong, level-headed Appalachian Trail walker I went through training with, as well as a black-haired, brown-eyed, twenty-two-year-old named Megan, who four years ago was herself a student in this same sweep of desert. Megan seems remarkably shy, reserved; talking with her I get the feeling she's on a kind of hero's path, struggling with a job that's likely to take her where she needs to go, but that on a lot of days carries with it a powerful sense of uneasiness, a challenge to her sense of self. Given the raucous nature of some of the kids, I wonder how she manages to keep from getting run over. Yet in the coming weeks even the most rambunctious of the girls will seek her out in some quiet setting, sit face to face in a wash or on a slab of sandstone pouring her heart out, as if only with Megan was it safe enough to be openly afraid.

On staff as well is Jonathan, a trim, muscular man of twenty-five with long, curly dark hair, a former professional dancer, calm as the dawn, full of seeking. And finally the senior instructor for the week—Josh, thoughtful and bemused. The son of the man who founded one of the most respected therapeutic boarding schools in the country, Josh has never known a life without troubled teenagers in close orbit. Two weeks from now he'll be gone from this desert, heading east to help found a new school for troubled teens in the hills of Massachusetts. Tonight when the girls flare up at one another Josh seems to take it all in stride; I can't really tell, though, if his reaction is that of a man who's really calm or merely tired.

Around the fire, between bites of spaghetti with red sauce and flour cakes cooked in the ashes, the girls go around and introduce themselves, recounting their litany of drug use and truancy and running away and "explosive episodes," as Jenna describes her last several years. Tricia, a perky, incredibly chatty fourteen-year-old from Ohio, tells how shocked she was to end up here—says even her parents thought this was going to be something like camp. "I show up with this big trunk filled with Clinique Face Wash and bottles of shampoo, all kinds of clothes," she says. "Next thing I know I'm at base being strip-searched by some lady, squatting so she can check to see if I'm hiding any drugs." She says they gave her a sandwich and made her drink a quart of water, which left her having to pee so badly on the car ride out to the field that, in a move I'll soon come to understand is classic Tricia, she persuaded the other three students with her to say they had to go too and then led the whole bunch of them in a begging chorus for a bathroom. The escort, a local fellow named Dallas, nodded quietly and drove them to an outhouse. Of course it was dark, and the outhouse didn't have any lights, so Tricia made him go in with a flashlight to make sure there weren't any spiders lurking about. "Back when I was a mouse," she tells me, making it sound as if it was in another lifetime, which in a way it was, "I was really homesick. Mostly, though, I was in shock."

For my part I tell the girls that some of why I'm here is because when I was their age, going through my own stuff, nature was the one place I could go to get my act together, where nobody judged me. That I'm a nature writer who's never gotten over being curious about the power of wild places. I offer a thanks for letting me hang out with them, and Tricia gives me a big smile filled with braces and asks if I'm going to make them famous.

After group tonight around the fire Nancy says that being a writer I surely must know some stories, and if that's the case I need to tell some. The other girls chime in, showing the kind of enthusiasm I would've thought more appropriate to walking down the road and finding a cooler full of Cokes and Snickers bars dropped off the back of a motor home. It's the first hint I have of what makes for one of the deepest pleasures out here— fire, mixed with just about anything kind to the imagination.

The story that pops into my head first is an old Ojibwa tale about the son of the West Wind, a creator named Nanabush; I scootch up close to the flames, take a breath, try to make the telling a gift.

It was a long time ago in the land of trees. Spirit Woman had given birth to human twins. Every animal was fond of those twins, always fussing over them, eager to keep them safe, make them warm and happy. Dog, for one, never left their side. Sometimes flies would pester the babies and Dog would snap at them to drive them away. Dog made them laugh by nuzzling their soft bellies with his nose, by jumping into the air and doing all kinds of tricks. When the twins got hungry Wolf and Deer gave their milk, and Bear kept them warm with his thick coat

*of fur. The birds sang them to sleep. Beaver washed them
in the lake.*

*But over time it dawned on the animals that some-
thing wasn't quite right. "We feed them, care for them,"
said Bear. "But they don't stand. They don't run and play
like our children do. The son of the West Wind, Nanabush, will come soon. We must ask his help." A few days
later, when Nanabush arrived, the animals told him their
worries. Nanabush listened carefully. He told the animals
they'd cared for the babies well. Too well. "Children grow
by reaching, striving for what they want," he said. "Not
by having everything placed in their laps. I will go and
ask Great Spirit what to do."*

*So Nanabush left the woods and went high into the
hills rising in the west. There he asked the Great Spirit
for help. Great Spirit heard the problem and he told Nanabush to scour the slopes of the hills for a certain kind
of sparkling stone. "Gather all you can find," he said.
"Then place them in a pile on the highest hill." So that's
what Nanabush did, collecting those colored stones, one
by one, until he had an enormous pile of them—fifteen,
maybe twenty feet high. But what next? Hour after hour
he sat there, hoping for some clue from Great Spirit, but
none came. Finally, out of boredom Nanabush sat down
beside the pile of stones, started tossing them into the air,
first one at a time, then several. One time he tossed a big
handful high into the air and they didn't come back
down again! Instead they changed into the most beautiful winged creatures—the very first butterflies.*

*Nanabush went back to the babies in the forest, sur-
rounded by a flashing, fluttering blanket of butterflies.*

The twins were delighted. They set about waving and stretching, trying to catch one in their chubby hands. For a long time they crawled after them, then stood on their tiny feet and tottered, and finally ran through the forest, laughing, all the while hoping to catch even one of those beautiful creatures.

And that, say the Ojibwa, is how butterflies taught children to walk.

The girls want another story, so I offer one from Java, "The Forest and the Tiger," and then they want another still, so I tell one from Africa called "The Coming of Darkness." On it goes, story after story, until finally we have to call an end to it because the firewood is gone and it's surely past midnight. I slip into my bag and stare up at a sky plumb full of stars. Nearby are the sounds of Susan sobbing, Tricia snoring, Jenna mumbling. It suddenly dawns on me that there's no place on earth I'd rather be.

The next morning is cold and clear, the frost so bright in the morning sun that the desert looks lit from within. Today is Tricia's fifteenth birthday, and Kristine is up just after dawn, wrapping herself against the chill in a wool blanket, making Tricia a batch of pancakes. After breakfast four of the girls blindfold Susan, the sad girl I picked up at the airport, and walk her down to Yarrow Springs, where they sit in a circle and one at a time say what being a mouse is all about, what the next couple of days are going to look like. Jenna tells her to hold out her hand, and she lays a piece of leather cordage in her palm. "It's a necklace," Jenna says. "There aren't any beads on it yet. It's empty to remind you the time has come to begin adding new things to your life." Then the girls tell her some of the rules: No future information given out; every night a buffalo or an eagle will collect her pants and shoes and leave them with staff; she'll need to ask staff to go to the bathroom and then count while she's out there taking care of business; as a mouse she can't talk or otherwise hang out with the rest of the group, and they won't be able to talk to her. "Other than on solo there won't be another time when you'll be able to be by yourself like this," Lisa says. But while that may seem like a good thing to Lisa, to Susan, wrestling with her depression, I wonder if being alone will be just another weight. By the time we walk back to camp she looks dejected—tired and hump shouldered. Lifeless.

An hour is spent crushing coals from the campfire with rocks and scattering them in the desert, loading the blue-tarp packs and the Dutch oven into the carts, centering and bracing the 150-pound water containers so they don't shift on these rugged roads. By 10:30 we're on the move, heading downhill, bound for who knows where. The conversation between the girls roams the known universe—boys, of course, and how Diet Dr Pepper is better than Diet Coke and Snapple is better than either; movies and amusement parks and people snoring; about Lavoy being the bomb. That Tricia definitely has the worst-smelling farts of anyone here. And for some, how scary it is to think of going home. There's definitely a sense of unity among the girls, especially those who've been here several weeks or more, and it goes well beyond misery loving company. It's equal parts resignation and confidence—a mix born out of the simple knowledge that they can and will spend this entire day grunting and groaning behind a pair of 500-pound carts and then bust out a hot meal and a decent place to sleep, and in the end that's vastly more satisfying than bitching about the fact that they have to do it at all. Watching them, I'm reminded of something I read once about how Eskimo are sometimes referred to as the most adult people on earth—that the climate is so harsh it takes tremendous maturity to keep going, to keep the community intact. Granted this is no trip across the ice floes. Still, in the good moments, I'm not so sure there isn't some honest-to-god adulthood leaking through.

A mile or so from Rabbit Butte we pass a couple of acres of yucca plants. When Josh tells the girls the root can be boiled and made into shampoo they all but beg to stop long enough to wrestle a few pieces from the ground with sticks and give it a try. Even lunch seems of minor importance next to the yucca harvest. We make camp an hour later, some six miles down the road from where we started this morning. Two of the girls get wood while Kristine, who calls herself the mother hen, busts out a bow-drill fire in less than thirty seconds, places three billy pots of water around the edges, tosses in the yucca roots, and prays for shampoo. Meanwhile fifteen-year-old Lisa, though she's living in the midst of what seems like an incredibly mellow staff, is having trouble with authority again—an alligator she's been wrestling for years. She sits with Josh, trying her best to yank his chain, and she's good at it. She complains that the staff treats the group as if they're guilty until proved innocent, that they go around expecting lousy behavior, that they should quit acting like parents and start acting like friends. She fairly bristles at the power they have over her.

"Look," I overhear her saying. "The thing is, most people don't question enough. Are you trying to tell me that questioning things isn't a part of living a good and purposeful life?"

"Not at all," Josh is saying, looking as if he's met his match. "But sometimes you have to make a leap of faith. None of us

are out here doing this job because we get a kick out of coming
down on you. This isn't some kind of power trip. We're trying
to create an atmosphere where things can happen for you,
where you'll get stronger. I can't prove that to you. It's something you're going to have to trust."

The hair washing is a major hit and leaves everyone in a
great mood. Even Lisa gives it a rest. Nancy and Carla decide to
engineer a pizza in the Dutch oven, loaded with onions and
cheese and tomato sauce, and afterward Kristine manages to
knock out a great birthday cake for Tricia, complete with chocolate frosting, a treat brought in by staff for every birthday. The
cake gets carried to the edge of the fire on a slab of sandstone,
accompanied by strains of the birthday song, is cut into pieces
with a Green River Knife, placed on sheets of notebook paper,
and handed out to everyone, staff and students alike. On finishing her piece of cake, Kristine—a girl who at various times can
take on the air of a southern belle—stuffs her piece of notebook
paper into her mouth, explaining to me that this is how she
cleans the last morsels of goodies from wax-paper cupcake hold-
ers, chews it for a while, then spits the wad into the fire. Everyone thanks Tricia for having a birthday. Then they get busy
counting the days left until the next one rolls around.

Late in the evening, with stars blazing overhead and the
fire burned to embers, Lisa and Jenna begin beating on the billy
pots, grunting out the rhythms and strange web of guttural
sound effects necessary to launch their "home girls" rap, which
has become pretty much a staple of Group 3. Games are played.
There are long, fresh peals of laughter. And for one sweet evening it does in fact seem nearly as if this is the experience Tricia
was expecting all along—a good time with new friends at summer camp. Complete with yucca shampoo.

CHAPTER FOUR

MATTERS OF LOVE AND GRAVITY

THE NEXT MORNING dawns clear, flawless. Full-spectrum lighting as only an April sun over a Southwest desert can provide. Meadowlarks and Western bluebirds flit about the junipers— every one of them, the Paiute would say, still wearing the bright colors of the beadwork that once decorated their buckskins back in the days when they were human. I'm especially pleased about the weather today because in a couple of hours the kids will be heading out on solos. And while rain and snow may have their own gifts to offer, right now I like the thought of them being able to sprawl out in the warm sand, write and sleep and putter, for one afternoon have the world go back to kid time, slow and thick and full of light.

During their eight-week stay in the wilderness the kids can expect to go through two solos, each lasting about two days and nights. Some blossom in the chance to care for themselves, feed on the sense of personal power that comes from being self-sufficient—knowing how to get warm, cook, stay dry. Dave, our trainer, tells how on a cold day in December he was making rounds of solo sites, quietly checking on students so as not to disturb them, when he found a fourteen-year-old boy standing in his underwear in front of a six-foot fire, arms crossed, looking very much like Yul Brynner in *The King and I*. "I'm not sure what happened," the boy confessed later, sheepishly. "I had all this wood around so I just kept putting more and more on, and suddenly it was huge."

The students don't know solos are happening until they're circled up and the staff suddenly tells them to undo their survival packs, take out all the food, and put it in a pile. And that's how it plays out this morning. We spend an hour reviewing the rules of solo and talking about its meaning, floating notions about what good might come of it. Some of the girls—leaders like Kristine and anarchists like Carla and Lisa—smile at the announcement, no doubt seeing solo as much needed relief from this crazy, rambling family of theirs. (There is one big negative for Carla, though. She reminds us that there are cows cruising around this place, talking about them as if they were bovine bandits, plotting, waiting until she's alone to barge onto her site and terrorize her. Josh tells her that if they come close she should just get up and walk away, but she takes no comfort from that. "What if I'm too afraid to move?" she asks.)

Other girls, though, the buddy-style talkers and the social butterflies, those with more serious ADD's, are unsettled by the thought of being alone with no one to talk to. ("We send a kid out on her own for a couple of days," as Lavoy put it, "and then see if she enjoys the company.") Tricia and Sara are upset nearly to tears. In truth, living in a culture where prolonged silences are virtually unknown, where we'll do damn near anything to fill up the blank spaces with noise, theirs seems the more normal reaction. Remarkably, by the time they've put on their blindfolds and we've walked them off to their sites, which are located anywhere from fifty yards to a quarter-mile from camp, even the most reluctant seem resigned to the experience. "Nothing I can do about it," Tricia tells me. "I'm gonna go on solo whether I'm mad about it or not." For the third time in twenty minutes she makes me promise to tell Pam, the therapist, to come by her site, a request that has less to do with her needing counseling than with an eagerness to get all the birthday mail she's sure is heading her way.

Shortly after we break the circle, Kristine, who herself came here with bulimia, comes up to Megan and Jonathan with some startling news about Nancy, saying that yesterday she confessed she's been throwing up pretty much every day since she got here. This is definitely not good news for someone about to go on solo, where it couldn't be easier to purge any time you want. A quick staff huddle, at which it's decided that Megan will go talk to Nancy, try to get all this out in the open, see if she's willing to come up with a plan for getting the support she needs. The two end up talking for a good hour. Megan tells her she understands what's going on, can sympathize, that right before she came here as a student four years ago she was waltzing with a major eating disorder of her own, starving herself, stemming her hunger with a fair amount of speed.

Given how difficult it is to provide moment-by-moment supervision in a wilderness setting, this program, like most others, tries to screen out kids with severe eating disorders. On the other hand, some staff claim they've seen few girls without some sort of eating problem. Sometimes parents decide not to mention that their son or daughter is dealing with such things simply because they're desperate to get them in. Other times, as in Nancy's case, her folks aren't even at the point where they're able to acknowledge their daughter's bulimia is real. When she was in sixth grade they enrolled her in a popular commercial diet program, which "sort of worked," as Nancy puts it, but only for a little while. And it was nothing compared to the solution offered by one of her friends in the seventh grade, who showed her how to stick her finger down her throat and get rid of calories as fast as she took them in. Now here she is, three years later, throwing up her oatmeal and beans and rice behind some rock in the middle of the Utah desert.

Nancy not only comes clean but musters enough courage to ask if someone could sit with her for an hour after she eats— the real danger zone for throwing up. She says it also helps if she exercises, so Megan suggests to Josh a plan that would allow the breaking of solo once a day to team up with either her or Elizabeth to go for a run. "None of this is anything we could just come out and tell her we were going to do," Megan tells me. "Bulimia is all about control. If we would've just handed that plan to her, she would've found a way around it." The staff huddles and talks the situation out, but only for a minute or two. They know such an approach will compromise the benefits of the solo experience, but obviously right now the bulimia is by far the bigger fish to fry. Josh gives the plan the okay, and with that Jonathan and Elizabeth blindfold Nancy and lead her up Magpie Wash to her site.

Back at camp Josh and I sit in the sand among the piñon

and junipers, spend some time just talking. He's having a rough time of it this week, trying to balance his compassion for the girls, be there for them, with the need to enforce the rules. Things have been especially strained with Lisa and Kristine, and given the force of their opinion with the rest of the group, it's causing stress at every turn. He says you can't be in charge out here without getting morphed into whatever male authority figure the girls have issues with at home: fathers, brothers, uncles, teachers. I ask him if he ever wonders if he cares too much. If the passion that draws him to the work might also leave him inclined to shoulder all the bad things that have happened in the girls' lives.

"I suppose that's true," he says. "For now I'm holding on to something that Pam tells us all the time: 'Sometimes you can be their friend. But what you have to be first is their guide.' "

Meanwhile Susan, still on mouse and therefore not going on solo, isn't doing well. She seems to be shrinking, closing in on herself, as if whatever breath of confidence there is that inspires people to normal size was leaking away. The problem is at its worst whenever she's by herself, and being alone is what the mouse phase is all about—trying to figure out why you're here, how you might plug yourself in. All the girls say that being a mouse is the toughest part of the entire program—sitting on the outside looking in, stewing in your own stuff, wondering over and over again how you ended up here. Susan's alone time is probably even more intense with the rest of the group out on solos, since she can't distract herself by eavesdropping on other conversations, can't lose herself in other lives.

To make matters worse, she's not drinking water. In arid country that's bad news for anyone, the cause of headaches and sore muscles and fatigue. But Susan is on a derivative of lithium, and lack of water can lead to kidney damage. Josh calls the problem in to Sandy, the nurse at base, and she says to tell Susan that if she doesn't get the water down on her own she'll have to come out and give it to her intravenously. Thankfully that does the trick. From then on Susan drinks like a fish, informing us with no small amount of pride whenever she finishes off another quart. It isn't always that way, Sandy will tell me later. Sometimes the warning backfires. Some kids, it seems, find a certain appeal in the thought of an IV needle stuck into their arm.

In the end Josh and the rest of the staff don't press the alone-time part of being a mouse all that hard with Susan, figuring that a time out is far more critical for someone full of rage than for someone full of nothing. When we talk I notice the slightest glint in her eye, as if conversation meant belonging, and in the belonging, at least a hint of hope. As soon as I leave, though, she crumples again. Heading off with Elizabeth to check on solo sites I look over my shoulder to see she's crawled back under her wool blanket, trying to sleep away the world.

The staff gathers early in the evening for a dinner of potato soup. Before we eat, Josh, Jonathan, Megan, and Elizabeth talk it over and decide to get Susan out of her bag, bring her over to hang out with us for a while. This time she's reluctant, as if she doesn't want to lose the comfort of being unconscious; finally she sits up, wipes the hair out of her face, puts on her glasses, grabs her blanket, and shuffles over and sits down next to the cook fire. Jonathan asks her about the time she spent in the hospital, in the suicide ward, where she was until just a few days ago. "I know all the rules by heart," she says, sounding grateful for the chance to tell her story. "See, they give you this little yellow book, the rules are all in there. Like no sharps"—

she says, falling fast into the lingo—"nothing you could hurt yourself with. When my mom brought me flowers, she had to put them in a plastic Coke bottle." She tells us how she couldn't go outside, that in fact the only hint of the outside was a screened-in patio in the adult ward, built for smokers. "I didn't spend much time there—it just made me depressed that I couldn't go out. Especially on nice days."

She talks about how the priest from her school came to see her, but thinks the priest from the family church came only because her dad pleaded with him. "He's not the kind to come to a place like that on his own," she explains, chafed about it. "My church cares only about the adults with money, not the kids. It's so stupid. I mean, eventually the kids are going to be the adults with money." She goes on for another twenty minutes, telling us in great detail about bed checks, about the lousy food, about John, the guy who broke the lock on the back door of the suicide ward and no one even knew about it—how he'd disappear for thirty minutes at a time, go off and meet a buddy out in the street who'd bring him bags of pot.

Late afternoon brings clouds—cold and gray, like they were spun out of steel; while so far the most they've managed here in the desert is a few drops of rain, from the looks of it they're loosing no end of fresh snow on Thousand Lake Mountain. Just when we're sure the storm is going to get us after all, two big fingers of blue sky crack open in the west to light a band of mist lying along the massive domes of Capitol Reef, turning them into sun-drenched turrets and ramparts, one minute half hidden and the next rising out of the gray like portals in the mists of Avalon. It's simply incredible, a show of beauty that completely overwhelms us, and before long Megan and Jonathan are running back and forth across the hills around camp, gaining this rise and then that one, trying to see it from every possible angle. In the last of the light a rainbow begins to form barely a half mile away, one end planted at the base of Rabbit Butte and the other just to the east, in the foothills of the Henrys. It comes in stages, a few weak bands at first, swelling to something fat, complete, every color clear, as if it had been finger painted on the sky. Even Susan, who by now has shuffled back to her bag, once more sad and dejected, comes hurtling out from under her tarp. "Wow! That's the biggest rainbow I've ever seen in my life!" she says, grinning for the first time in two days.

Near the end of the show Jonathan, Susan, and I stand together in a field of sage, a fresh, earth-scented wind fingering the grasses at our feet. For a long time we're quiet. Then Jonathan begins telling about his life as a professional dancer in Montreal. When Susan asks if he's ever hurt himself, he offers a curious, even outrageous response, telling her how over the years he's learned to equate gravity with love. "Every trip, every stumble, I remind myself that I'm merely falling into the arms of the earth. And so falling is no longer a scary thing." Susan looks a little confused, suspicious at first, as if he might be pulling her leg, but when it's clear he's not she seems amused, content to roll the thought around in her head for a while, savor it. Watching her, I can't help but think of the incredible transition she's made in the past seventy-two hours. From the halls of a suicide ward with her little yellow rule book, kept from having even her tape player lest she decide to strangle herself with the cord, staring out through the screens of an old smoker's lounge. And now, watching rainbows firing across some of the biggest skies in America, sleeping under a tree in the dirt, having someone tell her that when gravity is love there's no danger in falling.

Solos are meant to be a quiet time, so few words get traded between kids and staff. Whatever needs the girls have, from sunscreen to tampons, are shared by way of notes left at small rock piles, or cairns, located at the edges of their sites. This is also where staff leaves food—oatmeal and peaches and granola for breakfast, beans and rice and noodles for dinner, the latter to be cooked over a bow-drill fire. It's the talking in whispers with Elizabeth as we make the rounds, the occasional brief smile traded through the junipers with the girls who choose to make eye contact with us, and, most especially, the careful sifting of food from the palm of my hand into the cups waiting by those rock cairns, round after round, morning and night, that for me brings a certain beauty to solo, that turns this from a mere time out into something that feels close to sacred.

Carla is a particular joy to see, having fully embraced the idea of being one with the dirt. When we pass by in the evening I see her sitting in the sand, face smudged, writing poetry; the next morning she's drawing in her journal with a piece of left-over charcoal from her fire.

Jenna, on the other hand, who hates solos, apparently hasn't changed her mind. When we come by she either turns her back on us or sneers. And then there's Kristine—beautiful, stately Kristine—undisputed leader of the group. Kristine has excavated a sizable hole in the sand and lined it with tarps; each day she patiently heats cans of water on her fire and dumps them into the basin, creating a kind of ruffian's hot tub. On one of our rounds she comes over and greets us, army-green T-shirt and smoky sun-lit face, hair piled into a loose bun with a tampon sticking out above her ear, barefoot in the sand, brown eyes shining. Queen of the desert. Debutante at the Lord of the Flies ball.

Therapists for this program are responsible for one group, or roughly eight kids. Twice each week they make their way over trails and up washes, sometimes hiking with the group, talking with each kid as they walk; other times huddling for hours, going one-on-one in the shade of a cliff or under the branches of a cottonwood. Group 3's therapist is Pam, a fit, thirty-something workaholic who offers her charges a passionate, slightly eclectic mix of modern therapeutic technique and Sufi wisdom. Of all the therapists she's the only one who has been an instructor, which goes a long way in helping her know what the field staff is going through out here; she's quick to sense burnout and, probably just as important, willing to go to bat for the instructors when changes dreamed up at corporate head-quarters—like the push a few months back for strict staff dress codes—threaten their ability to make connections with the kids. "It's about nature, and it's about group dynamics—living to-gether twenty-four hours a day. But if I had to narrow it down, pick one thing that's really magic, it's the relationship that hap-pens between the students and the instructors." I've heard other therapists make the same comment. It leaves me thinking that this would be the worst job in the world for psychologists in the habit of being territorial, especially when that territory ends up being shared with a group of mildly off-center twenty- and thirty-somethings who drive old cars and sleep on people's floors.

Pam's approach to working with kids seems less a matter of prescription than discovery. That, along with her willingness to huddle under a tarp in a downpour, or dine with the kids on a few bites of burned beans at ten o'clock at night, is what prompts a lot of these girls—even those who say they hate therapists—to feel at ease with Pam, to trust her. At least on their better days.

Not that therapy around here is some kind of love fest. "We've been therapisized to death," Lisa and Jenna have told me, echoing a sentiment shared by so many of the kids who end up at programs like this. "It sucks," as Jenna put it. "We're sick to death of it. Tell them what they want to hear, and hope they leave you alone. I guess Pam's not so bad, though." Still, as liaisons between kids and their parents—coaxing out letters and personal contracts to deal with critical family issues, calming anguished moms and dads during weekly phone calls—these therapists too can sometimes be seen by the kids as Mom and Dad's hired guns. Besides, it's largely on the recommendation of the therapist that parents may decide that what Jane or Johnny faces back at home isn't going to be healthy—that after completing this program they should go on to aftercare, which usually means some kind of therapeutic boarding school.

Not going home is a constant source of conversation, especially among the girls. A couple days ago I heard Jenna asking Kristine what she'd do if her parents told her they weren't going to let her come home. "I'd run," Kristine said with a steely look. "I would. I'd just start running." Which launched Jenna into a grand fantasy in which she dresses up all proper, drives into

Loa, and says she's Kristine's mom, and the two of them climb
in the car and speed off to California. Tricia, never far from the
action, looked more than a little panicked when eyes turned to
her. "Look, dude, my mom wrote and told me how she's redec-
orating my room for when I get back. My grandma said she's
baking me a cake. Man, I'm going home!"

Pam arrives, as usual toting a backpack full of mail. Since the
kids have no phones to lean on, the art of letter writing thrives
here—not just as a means of sharing the stuff of daily life, but
as a safe, deliberate way to convey the heavy, heartfelt feelings
that neither child nor parents were ever able to say to one another back home. It begins with the first rendering by parents
of why they felt they had to send their kids here—so-called
impact letters—handwritten notes, mailed or faxed, then tossed
into a daypack and carried to the desert. As the weeks go on,
feelings of rage and betrayal, and later, at least for some, feelings
of sadness and regret—the owning of the past and the hoping
for the future—all get traded through the written word.

Now and then—like today—the pages turn heavy. Enough
bad news in Pam's daypack to send our little tribe into a frenzy,
words from home that will make my days until now with Group 3
seem like a holiday with the Brady Bunch.

Less than a week ago, in what she clearly considers an act
of courage, Kristine wrote a letter to her dad, calling him on
some questionable behavior—comments she thought had sexual
overtones, walking in on her in the bathroom, taking her out to
the bars and leaving Mom at home. He's written back, sounding
terribly formal, saying he can't believe she'd think such a thing.
And then the last paragraph—the worst part—the part that says

when this program is over Kristine won't be coming home.

Four or five years ago, the relatively few kids who went to aftercare would find out about it only a couple of days before graduation. As often as not that just wasn't enough time for them to get a handle on their rage. Sometimes those kids would walk out of the wilderness at graduation and spit on their parents, curse them, turn their backs, and refuse to speak. Now such news tends to get delivered well in advance, giving the kid a chance to try to work through it with her group.

Those of us back at camp can tell it hasn't gone well long before we hear it from Pam. Long before she has a chance to tell us about Kristine getting aggressive in a way she'd never seen before, cursing her, coming within inches of throwing punches. We know because we can hear the wailing rolling through the darkness—great, heaving sobs pushing up Magpie Wash into the smoke of our cook fire, drifting out to the other solo sites scattered about in these dark huddles of juniper.

I forget for a minute that Kristine is an eagle, and that one of the privileges of an eagle is carrying a Green River Knife, and when Josh brings it up, for a split second I feel sick. Pam doesn't think it's a problem, but to be safe she asks Josh and Megan if they'd go back to Kristine—just be there for her; the two grab a couple of water bottles, and thirty seconds later they disappear into the trees, walking fast toward the sound of crying.

Pam takes a few swigs from a water bottle, wipes her mouth with the back of her hand, and moves off through the woods to deliver yet another load of dynamite, this one to Sara, with the same, awful message about not going home. Sara is one of the most original, compelling kids you could ever hope to meet. Of all the girls, she's completely taken with the notion that being dirty is a badge of honor. On most days her hair looks like it was combed with a blender, and her face and legs and arms are three sheets of gray, about how you'd expect somebody to look after a week spent shoveling coal. The look seems a strength.

Sara's been diagnosed as bipolar, which means that on most days she's either full of joy or quiet and withdrawn. Unlike Susan, though, she doesn't seem the least bit inclined to collapse under the weight of it. Even on her darkest days she'll grit her teeth and squeeze the depression into something like anger, riding the tail of that emotional whirlwind until she stumbles out on the other side. And when she gets there, there isn't one of us who doesn't feel somehow as if a bit of her strength has landed in our pockets. But the weight of the news about not going home seems to undo her. Even though she knew when she came that this would probably be a stop on the way to another program, a school of some sort, there was still that measure of hope—that little kid in there, wanting and hoping to go home.

For all her quirkiness, there's one thing that makes Sara as common as a spring wind, though, and that's having been a kid who's controlled her family for a very long time. While she's been out here wrestling with her stuff, her parents have been back in Boise doing therapy twice a week, building the resolve to make contracts with their daughter and stick to them, to write the rules and enforce them—to be parents instead of friends. Attempting to reorder the power structure with a kid past the age of nine or ten, say many therapists, is guaranteed to be a struggle of near mythic proportions. It was never a matter of neglect, Sara's parents will tell me when I see them at her graduation. It wasn't that she took over the family because everyone else was too busy doing their own thing. It was that her illness, her depression, made them sad, and what they wanted more than anything in the world was for her to be happy. That the happiness could come at the cost of her character, her sense of self, was something that never occurred to them.

With Josh and Megan off to spend time with Kristine, Jonathan and Elizabeth head out to help Nancy get a bow-drill fire so she can eat hot, then sit with her for a while so she isn't tempted to throw it up. Susan and I can't stay alone together at camp (a single staff person is never allowed to be alone with a student) so the two of us tag along, hang out at the far edge of Nancy's solo site under a cluster of junipers. We talk about some of what she needs to do in order to move out of the mouse phase, which includes coming up with why she's here, as well as what she can offer the group. "I can cook," she tells me with certainty. "I'm good at it, too. And I'm rational, a problem solver. I can help the group find solutions to whatever things might come up."

She talks about her mom, a social worker—Susan is really proud of her—about her sister and brother, her dad the accountant. She lays out a couple of thoughts on how she ended up here, what went wrong. "I guess it started back in junior high, seventh grade. The kids were always teasing me, making fun of me. I didn't fit in. Last summer I started fantasizing about suicide—I'd imagine my funeral, who would be there, what they'd say. Stuff like that." She says a few months ago she started self-mutilation, cutting herself, and that was right before her second trip to the suicide ward. "I don't know. I imagine it must be a way of punishing myself for something."

We sit for more than two hours, the night growing steadily colder, until I have to run back to camp to get her a couple of wool blankets to keep away the chill. Through much of the evening we're down on our knees, under the big trees, nose to the ground, looking for brown, pea-size juniper seeds that have been pierced on one side by a certain hungry insect. Ghost beads, they're called. Perfect for stringing onto sinew for necklaces and bracelets. One somewhat Anglo-sounding story tells of the need to have 101 ghost beads as you pass from this world into the next—one as a gift for each of the hundred warriors who guard the gates of the hereafter, and one extra, just in case Coyote, the trickster, shows up. I can't say much about the power of ghost beads in the next life, but they definitely have something special going for them in this one. If food is a kind of substitute for money out here, ghost beads, for whatever reason, are for many the ultimate in personal possessions. As the months unfurl I'll see the strange magic of gathering ghost beads shine through time and again: salve for the angry, comfort for the depressed, play for the hopeless, and perhaps most remarkable of all, one more thing that kids with even severe ADD are able to focus on with barely a hint of fidgeting.

Megan and Josh come back from Kristine's site, having spent the first hour helping her vent, then the next encouraging her to imagine life beyond a therapeutic boarding school. It was rough, they tell us, even scary. "I've got two options," she told them when they arrived at her site. "Life or death. Right now I don't know which is better." Over time, though, she calmed down, and toward the end managed to summon a striking defiance—one suggesting that absolutely no one was going to beat her.

Kristine is the first to admit that she's a merciless self-critic. Exactly like her mother. Deep down she thinks people in therapeutic boarding schools are broken, damaged goods—just as she once thought about kids here. And the fact is it's not okay for her to be tossed into a school full of imperfect people. Besides, she argues, putting her in a therapeutic boarding school is a terrible idea because of the heavy structure of such places. "Push me into a corner, and I'll end up going right back to my old ways. My bulimia. That's how I cope." On hearing that, Josh asks her if she needs to exercise here on her site as a means of dealing with her stress. She tells him she has to be careful, that too much exercise will trigger her desire to purge.

"After two-and-a-half years I still hate this part of the job," Pam says after finishing her rounds sometime shortly before midnight, looking weary, beaten down. She asks how it went with Susan, and I tell her about our conversations, confess that it was good to see her so interested in something, even if it was only ghost beads. Pam says that Susan's having been suicidal twice over the past nine months makes her a marginal admission— points out that we'll have to keep a close eye on her, that she stands a good chance of being pulled from the program.

Next on Pam's agenda comes a thirty-minute meeting with staff about what issues to coax and what buttons to push in the week to come; then off to the side, with Josh, a reminder to not get caught up in Kristine's anger. "Remember," she says, zipping up her Gore-Tex, hefting her backpack, "Kristine is dealing with a lot of stuff right now, issues about her father. It may feel like she's going after you, but she's going after him."

It's a short, bitter night. Even the normally bubbly, silly Tricia is haunted by bad dreams. Dreams of being back in school and pulling somebody else's bag of crack out of her locker right as a bunch of cops come down the hall. "They spun me around and shoved me up against the wall so hard I could feel it in my sleep," she'll tell us when she comes off solo, looking troubled

even then. "What am I going to do when I get back? Every place
I want to go there's old friends, and all the drugs. They'll still
be there, just like before."

My dreams too, are strange, unsettling. The one I remember best is short—some guy coming to my home town with a
pen full of coyotes, wanting to use them as a tourist attraction.
My friends and I are incensed, end up running up Main Street
looking for an attorney to help us stop him.

We begin pulling people off solo around midafternoon, but only
after lengthy individual conversations with them, trying to get a
sense of how things went. Fourteen-year-old Carla, this being
the end of her first solo, is euphoric. When we arrive she's
sitting in the shade of a juniper writing in her journal. Beside
her is a pile of bones she's collected, a quart water bottle full
of juniper berries, and a rather impressive sand castle. She
shows Josh and me the *pawawka* she made after reading the
legend about Tecumseh, when he dived into that icebound
river, day after day, trusting that there was something to be had
from it that he could use on his journey into manhood.

"Inside the pouch," Carla tells us, "I put a Moqui marble,"
which is a local term for the small, round sandstones that cover
much of this desert. "It stands for the circleness of life, how life
goes either in expanding or contracting circles. You can go inward and end up in a tight, fetal position. Then the only way
out is back, one circle at a time, bigger and bigger, but slowly,
never all at once." Onto the outside of the leather pouch she's
fixed a piece of quartz, which she says represents her hope for
clarity.

"Do you think Tecumseh needed his brother there by his

side, lending support, to keep jumping in the river?" Josh asks her.

"Maybe at first he needed his brother's help," she says. "But after a while he probably was strong enough to do it on his own. If a *pawawka* is supposed to offer power," she continues, "then there's going to have to be some sort of ordeal involved in getting it. That's where my *pawawka* is different. It isn't so much about strength—it's about peace."

Carla's well aware that she doesn't fit in easily, here or anywhere else, being brilliant and a little dark, eccentric beyond her years. Some of the girls don't quite know what to do with her. The difference between Carla now and two weeks ago, Josh says, has to do with her newfound confidence—a willingness to be who she is and let the chips fall where they may. Sitting here in the sand, I ask her if she thinks that's true.

"Tuesday I got a letter from my dad," she answers. "He said my mother is the way she is because she can't help it. 'But you can help it, Carla.' That was like this bolt of clarity. I realized for the first time I could choose one way of being over another. That I've got control over what I do, who I am." Another letter came that day, too—one that may have had some push and power of its own. It was written to Carla on Passover, wishes stitched together by her entire family—uncles, aunts, cousins—all passing sheets of paper around the dinner table so everyone could tell her how much they were thinking of her, how much they missed her. "Even Uncle Jake wrote something," she tells me with an enormous smile. "He's so funny. I really love Uncle Jake."

She says she has something to show us, rummages through the small canvas bag students are given at the beginning of the program, brings out a knife sheath she's made. Sewn into the leather is a beautiful web design, complete with a spider crafted from a single red bead. It's from a vision she had on her first night of the solo, she explains, a picture of the last couple years spent protecting herself by being a terrific liar. She flips through the pages of her journal and finds a poem she wrote about it.

> I am the weaver.
> I have woven my webs of deceit,
> trickery, mistrust and belligerency
> these delicate threads
> spun all together—wisps in the wind
> sticky on your fingers
> shining like diamonds—false as can be.
>
> I am the weaver—a black widow spider
> threads cling close to the center,
> spreading out slowly to catch my prey.
> They twist and they turn with no way to go.
>
> I am the weaver.
> I have woven my webs.
> They have all been torn down or blown away by the wind,
> and I watch as they waft gently to the ground,
> lie noiseless and empty,
> fallen to pieces—ripped to shreds
> my webs have all disappeared
> leaving only me.

She packs up her gear, and as we turn to go she stops, looks back at a grandfather cottonwood tree that has literally gone from bud to leaf in the three days of her solo. "I came to this place, and I ended up staring at that tree for hours and hours. Somewhere in that I realized happiness is something to be found inside me."

Our next call—and this time I'm with Jonathan—is to Sara;

her reaction could hardly be more different: sharp, full of ice. She sits cross-legged, hunched over the letter from her mom and dad, teeth and fists clenched and daggers in her eyes, hating Pam, her parents. Hating us. Her trademark dirty look, instead of seeming spirited, now seems only to highlight her sense of having been abandoned, a throwaway waif sitting all alone in the sage and the cheat grass. Jonathan is slow, patient, trying to encourage her to talk it out, but gets absolutely nowhere.

"All this fucking therapy, I swear I've had it." Jonathan asks why she hates therapy, at which point she looks straight at him, tells him it's because of all the stupid questions, "just like you're asking now." Over the past two weeks, Jonathan says, he's felt like a brother to Sara, and he takes this outburst hard. When we get back to camp he asks Josh for some personal time and walks off up the bench, looking incredibly sad. "Grief carried on the wind," he writes in his journal. "Over juniper trees and blooming locoweed like a fragrance in the air that turns my stomach. I sit next to a heart like a pincushion turned inside out—stabbing her as she cushions us all."

By midafternoon everyone is back, and we circle up in the sand for a feelings check. Oddly, Kristine strolls in looking pretty much okay—not happy, but then not the rage-filled, red-eyed wreck I was expecting. "I'm still angry about having to go on from here," she tells the group. "But I'm glad to be here right now." Carla feels happy, Lisa feels anxious, Sara feels angry, and Nancy, referring to her weight, feels gross. Tricia is proud of herself that she made it through solo at all—says she used some of the time to write her mother a letter coming clean about all the drugs she'd done, telling her she wanted a fresh start. "Sitting around out there I figured out I'm not going to be pampered anymore." She tells us that when she gets out she and her mom are going to Narcotics Anonymous together. "She used to be an addict, too."

The cohesiveness of the group tends to be at its strongest after solo—assuming, that is, that you're a part of the group to begin with. And Susan is not. She sits outside the circle, head down, looking incredibly sad, listening as Lisa reads a piece of writing she says is a gift to the rest of the girls—a story about a reunion that happens years down the road, the seven of them reuniting (Susan would be number eight), coming back to the desert to relive this whole experience. Ironically, only minutes before the rest of the girls blindfold Susan to take her off for a transition ceremony, where she'll finally become a coyote, officially part of the group, she pulls Jonathan aside, nearly in tears. "Have you ever felt your soul was, like, dead?" she says. "And your body just wanted to follow?"

Most of the time the rituals offered during transitions are thoughtful, powerful, life affirming. Other times they're lame, uninspired. Susan's is closer to the latter—a ho-hum recounting of what it means to be a coyote, what the rules are, and then a fast break to fix dinner. Long after we eat, with nearly everyone else in bed, Susan sits with us and picks up where she left off with that earlier comment to Jonathan. She says she might hurt herself if she could, though she doesn't really see how that's possible out here. "It's like a whirlpool, and I'm caught in it. I want to get out but I can't."

"What's at the bottom of the whirlpool?" Jonathan asks her.

"I don't know. Death, I guess."

She tells us that at least at home, in the hospital, she could talk to her family, that her doctor was just a phone call away.

And that just when she's gotten used to us as staff, tomorrow the staff is changing, and she hates that. She asks if she can sleep with us again tonight, says she doesn't feel safe, which around here is another way of saying you've got a mind to hurt yourself. Josh decides to put her on suicide watch and reviews the procedures with the rest of the staff: collecting all the knives; taking her bootlaces; laying a tarp over her with one person on either side. I volunteer to sleep with the ax under my bag. Tomorrow we'll tell the group to begin shadowing her every move.

"This is a good thing," Jonathan says to me, perhaps catching a flicker of alarm on my face. "We knew she was borderline when she came. Now we can put our full attention into keeping her safe." In the morning Josh tells the group that Susan is on suicide watch, asks someone to review what that means. The whole time Susan sits there cross-legged, buckled over, using a stone to draw images of crosses in the sand. We wrap it up, begin packing to move again. Just another day on the job, even for those on suicide watch.

Right as we finish loading the carts, a truck approaches in the distance, stops several hundred yards from us, and Jenna gets out, back from a trip to the orthodontist to repair a broken set of braces. Of course everyone wants to know what she saw and did, hoping if not for news of the outside world then at least reminders of it. She talks of seeing people drinking Cokes and surprising the heck out of herself by not having the slightest desire for one, concluding that the wilderness must be turning her into some kind of health freak. "Hey, dude, catch this. I walk into this guy's office, the orthodontist—by the way, he's got the same exact name as my orthodontist at home, is that freaky or what?—anyway there are these two cute high school boys in the waiting room." Of course, she says, everyone is staring at her—the boys, the receptionist—what with her smudged face and ripped khaki pants covered with patches of wildly colored fabric sewn on with the same thick waxed filament used for necklaces and *pawawkas*. "Hey!" she shouts at them, as I'm sure only Jenna could do, sounding stern, probably also flashing the slightest grin. "Gimme a break! I'm from the wilderness program in Loa—we don't take showers!"

Shortly after leaving Magpie we come to a steep, blistering incline littered with rocks. The girls decide to work together, pushing the carts up one at a time. It's a phenomenal effort, as I find out when I get in the back to lend a hand. Josh has put Tricia and Sara together with Susan on the cart, a move I'm beginning to see was a master stroke. Tricia is by far the most judgmental and cliquish of the lot, and this is a chance for her to take Susan under her wing, which she does right away, engaging her in a nonstop barrage of banter.

When Tricia runs out of steam Sara starts up, comparing notes with Susan about their experiences in the suicide ward, what it's like to be bipolar, what lithium and Depakote do to your head. "It sucks to be depressed," Sara says. "My favorite thing in the world is snowboarding—I went when I was depressed and it was no fun at all."

"I know!" Susan agrees, wiping beads of sweat from her forehead. "Like I went into the hospital for depression. They had a limo come and take me out for dinner for my birthday. It was okay on the surface, but I couldn't enjoy it at all."

On they go, sweating up the desert road in ninety-degree heat, past fresh gardens of paintbrush and penstemon, blooms open now, reaching for the sun, breaking talk only when they have to grunt to get the carts up a hill. By noon Susan, the girl who two nights ago told me she's never fit in anywhere, seems to have found a place to fit in after all, however hard-core and godforsaken it might be.

We eat lunch, do a round of curriculum in a wash flanked by rippled sandstone, rimmed by junipers. Rising in the south and west is an extraordinary jumble of nut-colored cliffs and towers marking the eastern boundary of Capitol Reef National Park. Today's lesson is about meteors and comets, and the staff teaching it plucks stones from the bank of the wash and places them in orbit lines traced in a clean sweep of sand. If you didn't know what was going on you might think it was a lesson in prehistoric art, or even early religion, the stones meant to symbolize the people as they walk the rounded paths that Carla says make up the circles of our lives. Partway through the lesson Kristine suddenly announces that her new name should be Sirius, after the Dog Star, though for the life of her she can't say why.

We push on for another three hours before stopping for the night. Jonathan and I are walking together in the sweet light of a desert sunset, him telling me of an exquisite cooking spice from the Middle East called zatar, then launching into a cherished dream of his: to one day be able to walk off into a wilderness—he hasn't figured out which one, and wants my thoughts—stark naked, to live there on his own for a year or two, making his own clothes and getting his own food.

And suddenly it's Wednesday, staff change. Nancy is talking to Megan and Jonathan about her bulimia. "I don't know how much I want to stop throwing up. But you're all trying so hard. I don't want to let you guys down." In other words, she's eager to give it up for other people but is still lukewarm about giving it up for herself. The good news, I suppose, is that she's at least willing to try some changes. She and Megan spend the next half hour working out a plan for how she'll eat in the coming week. In an effort to encourage responsibility, a certain mindfulness, kids are required to consume everything they cook; not doing so can mean cutbacks the following week. A careless, over-generous cook at the helm can mean passing the pot of leftovers around the circle at the end of the evening for what is commonly called a "yum-yum," pulling together to make it all disappear. From now on, no yum-yums for Nancy. Also, she says she'll try to eat only certain foods for lunch, staying away altogether from granola, which is the one thing that most leaves her wanting to purge.

During circle-up at staff change Nancy sits cross-legged in the sand, fumbling with a twig, struggling for the nerve to talk about her bulimia in front of everyone. Some of her reluctance comes from the fact that she sees herself as caretaker of these girls; it's not easy to reverse roles, ask for help instead of give it. In the end, though, she does just that, explaining the new eating plan to the rest of the girls and telling them what they can do to support her. If nothing else, her coming clean seems to push Susan to go for some help of her own. "I tend to go off by myself when I start feeling bad," she tells the girls. "If you see me sitting alone, if you wouldn't mind just coming over and talking to me." We go around the circle and share our highs and lows for the week, and when it gets to Susan she says her low was coming here at all, and that she really didn't have any highs. Jonathan nudges her to think of how happy she was when she figured out how to make natural cordage out of yucca fiber, the good job she's done on the carts, other accomplishments. "Yeah," she says sadly. "I guess. But that's all stuff on the outside."

There are times when getting out of the wild after eight days and nights with the kids feels like stumbling ashore after a shipwreck, washing to safety after a week spent hugging a two-by-four through heavy seas. This is one of them. Josh, Jonathan, Elizabeth, and I make a fast stop at Wanda's Drive-Inn in Loa for deep-fried zucchini and candy bar milkshakes, toss on some better-smelling clothes, and rush over to a potluck at Paula's house in Bicknell. There's dancing to be had in the living room, and before he can finish stuffing a single corn chip into his mouth, Josh is out there gyrating on the carpet in the most amazing release of pent-up angst I've ever seen. Most amazing, at least, until Jonathan, the former gymnast and professional dancer, moves out onto the floor. I sit open-mouthed on the couch with a beer in my hand while he hovers and floats in his chi pants and tie-dyed T-shirt, finally launching into a staggering array of handsprings and backflips, his long wavy hair flying. Paula comes into the room from cleaning up in the kitchen and stands in the doorway with her breath held, praying, I suspect, that a misplaced kick doesn't break the lamps or knock over the bookcases. In truth nearly everyone who's just come off course is blowing off steam with such vigor I can't help but wonder what they must do when there's no Wednesday night potluck with a decent stereo. It also explains something I heard before training started—how all the sweet Mormon families living in these neighborhoods tend to freak at the thought of ending up next to a "program house."

CHAPTER FIVE

TENTS FULL OF ACORNS

YOU COULD JUST about argue that it was meant to be. A people who cut their teeth on nature, wresting from the woods of eastern America visions to kindle patriotism, art, even religion, ending up two hundred years later using wilderness to feed the souls of troubled teenagers. Even plain old organized camping, now nearly 150 years old, turned on the idea that one of the best ways for kids to ready themselves one day to lead meaningful, successful lives was to toss off the city now and then to go live in the woods. The Boy Scouts, the Girl Scouts, the Sons of Daniel Boone, and a host of other programs long since come and gone sprouted from no more than that.

But when it came to using nature for therapy, as a source

of healing—that we stumbled into without a clue. It was 1901. Dr. A. E. Macdonald, of the New York psychiatric facility Manhattan State Hospital East, found himself in the alarming position of having forty men and women with tuberculosis who needed to be isolated from the rest of the patients, and absolutely nowhere to put them. Serious trouble, made more so by the fact that most clinicians of the day thought mental patients were especially susceptible to tuberculosis. Finally, more out of desperation than inspiration, Macdonald decided to erect a handful of tents around the grounds and put the infected patients there. At which point he got a big surprise.

Not only the physical but the mental state of the patients improved dramatically. The same people who'd been lying in their beds in a near vegetative state were walking on the grass, playing games, smiling, and waving at the excursion boats cruising up the East River. Macdonald put up another tent, this one for nontubercular psychiatric patients, more than 60 percent so ill they couldn't get out of bed. It worked for them, too. They gained weight, showed increased control over their compulsions, stopped wetting the bed. Several who had been thought to be lost causes two months earlier were by autumn walking out the front door. Everything continued to go well until late in the year, when the weather changed and all but one of the tents came down. The patients headed back inside, where they withdrew again, resumed their bad habits, lost weight, and became incontinent. And they stayed that way until the following summer, when the tents went up again.*

*C. Floyd Haviland, M.D., and Chester Lee Carlisle, M.D., "Extension of Tent Treatment to Additional Classes of the Insane," *American Journal of Insanity* (July 1905), p. 100.

Physicians came running from all over that hospital. Drs. Floyd Haviland and Chester Carlisle applied the idea to patients about to be released—a group that often frustrated doctors by slipping back into old ways under the stress of dealing with going home. For them, too, the results were striking. "The beneficial effects of outdoor life can be judged," wrote the doctors, "when it is stated that out of the entire forty-four patients, there have been only three on continued medication during the summer."

Tent therapy, they called it—the beginning of a twenty-year movement that would spread across much of the country. Still more fuel got added to the fire when the 1906 San Francisco earthquake shook to rubble a sizable part of the Agnew Asylum for the Insane. Amid the wreckage a shell-shocked Dr. Andrew Hoisholt set about helping his patients erect temporary shelters out on the lawns with tents and lean-tos, prayed for the best, and then to his utter amazement found most of them doing a lot better out on the lawns living like nomads than locked up inside. "I was astonished," he wrote in the *Journal of Insanity*. "Men and women who had been more or less constantly violent and untidy in the building were now getting along peacefully. They all seemed more comfortable and contented in the tents and on the open grounds. The record of the patients' condition and conduct during this enforced outdoor life certainly speaks well for tent treatment."* Hoisholt went on to note that even the epileptics were having fewer attacks.

For all its success, by 1920 the tent therapy movement was fading. A lot of it had to do with that age-old American bad habit of thinking that if some is good, more must be better, which

---

*Andrew Hoisholt, M.D., Letter to the Editors, *American Journal of Insanity* 63 (1906), p. 131.

prompted directors to expand their tent programs to ridiculous levels. Soon after its founding, the Manhattan State Hospital East program swelled to 175 patients, with plans for 300. Eventually someone got tired of replacing the tents and built pavilions instead, and before long those became little more than extra wards, locked up and overcrowded just like their predecessors in the days of old. Gone was much of what experts later figured made the whole thing work in the first place—small, cohesive groups who were given not just fresh air, but a sense of adventure, play, and improvisation.

Still, it was to some extent what happened out on those lawns that in 1929 led to the founding of the first therapeutic camp for regular kids, Camp Ahmek. Ahmek's primary goal was the same as that of any other program for kids: Engage the campers. To that end they served the usual plate of interactive games, sports, and swimming, all the while selling—as were hundreds of social pundits of the day—a strong message about the dangers of kids giving up their own playtime to become watchers of accomplished athletes: "spectatoritis."

Camp Ahmek's second goal—and this is where the therapy kicked in—was to help campers learn to build relationships with one another, give them an understanding of the power of community. The natural setting was thought to be a perfect place to teach such lessons, since living in the outdoors tended to make the consequences of not getting along with others not only a whole lot more obvious and immediate, but more logical, too. Don't help get the tent up, it rains, you get wet. Then, as now, kids who'd come to lean on some rather lame coping skills—hiding out from people they didn't like, distracting themselves from important issues—ended up for the first time in their lives having to come up with alternatives.

Those who worked at such programs made frequent mention of how great a teaching aid it was to have nature in your face twenty-four hours a day. A kid couldn't "save up his troubles, tears, or tempers until he goes home," as one observer put it years later. "If he is to have satisfaction, consolation, praise, or triumph, he must find it with the campers and counselors."* As near as anyone can figure, then, it was right there at good old Camp Ahmek that modern mental health professionals rediscovered the ancient idea of letting nature itself, with its bugs and its winds and its storms, set the price for blowing relationships.

As time went by, therapeutic camping yielded a barrage of enthusiastic responses from staff and parents about improvement in children's levels of responsibility, school performance, and self-control. Yet even the most celebrated weren't doing the kind of empirical research that would make such results real to the powers that be, and thus ensure the flow of funding. (To be fair, the use of reliable standardized measures to track outcomes in any sort of psychotherapy—even the traditional kind, practiced with the patient on the couch—was rare as dry feet at canoe camp.) Good programs sprouted, flowered—some of them in the most wonderful ways—and then withered on the vine.

Part of it also had to do with the fact that most mental health leaders were inclined, as many are to this day, to squeeze what goes on in such programs into existing textbook theories instead of doing original work on-site. It was an approach that drove people like noted New York child psychologist Dr. Ernest Harms nearly to distraction. To Harms and others it seemed

*R. Backus, "Where the New Camping Tasks Begin," *The Nervous Child* 16 (1947), pp. 130–34.

ludicrous for a test psychologist to stop by camp for a few hours, do some quick interviews with the kids, then over lunch casually announce to the staff that what the bully down by the lake slapping little Johnny around needed most was to relax his superego.

Even today, the therapeutic directors of the best wilderness programs are perfectly able to cite the accepted theories their programs turn on (God knows they get enough practice, jumping through hoops for skeptical insurance companies): psychodynamics, cognitive therapy, behavior modification. At the same time many say such theories don't begin to address what really happens. As the therapeutic director for this program says, "My theories have been largely formed by my experience; what I believe now comes from having worked here."

Besides, some of what works in the sticks seems to fly in the face of what's accepted elsewhere. For starters, the notion at the heart of much of American psychology today—that a kid is the result of something, his upbringing, his genetics—is barely talked about, primarily because it paints the kids as victims right from the start. Far more common around these parts is to try to see dysfunction in terms of specialness, as a unique path or calling—a sign, as one therapist put it, of something new struggling to emerge. Sort of like Jungian analyst James Hillman's description of childhood being an acorn, and within that acorn, a whole oak tree. Dysfunction, he says, is sometimes simply due to the fact that the oak—the kid's potential—is just too big for him to carry.

"Does contemporary psychology give you any reason for being here?" Hillman once asked. "Isn't that what someone wonders about—what am I here for, what am I called to do?

We need to talk of our lives in terms of imagination, not our lives in terms of chromosomes."*

It's untidy as hell, loose ends lying all over the place. In truth we may never know why eating beans out of a billy can or making a bow-drill fire can bring comfort, why on one particular rainy morning a carpet of desert phlox, the sound of a mourning dove, would bring a kid to tears. Why a stray comment made on the side of a mountain can change a life, can root and grow in what a month before seemed like sterile soil. A lot of the good that goes on in a program like this seems due less to the application of existing theory than to a mixed bag of tactics and intuitive strategies, hand-delivered by a slightly freaky bunch of mentors, in a place a thousand miles beyond the frenzy of the culture at large.

*James Hillman, interview, "The Best of Our Knowledge," National Public Radio, June 1977.

CHAPTER SIX

KEROUAC AND HIS BAND OF THIEVES

AT LAST A shower, about four hours' sleep on Josh's floor, and I'm off again, this time to visit the boys of Group 4. Brad, therapist for the group, picks me up outside the Post Office around seven-thirty and we head east out of Bicknell, munching apples and making for the desert. "This Jeep," he says sheepishly, nodding at the dashboard. "I ordered the thing through a guy in California—didn't know until I'd had it almost a month that it wasn't four-wheel drive. I'm getting a lot of grief from staff about it." If you think that suggests a certain lack of outback savvy, be assured that Brad fits in well here. More important than his choice of car are his worn jeans and tennis shoes, the faded black baseball hat cocked sideways above his round, boyish-looking face. There's a realness, a genuineness to him, and he seems perfectly willing to show confusion, frustration, to agree that things aren't fair, to tell a kid he just doesn't know.

Brad says that in the fourteen months he's been here he's found his own sense of spirit growing, in no small measure thanks to how easy it is in this environment to focus on the big questions. East of Torrey he looks out the side window at the waves of stone running up the spine of Capitol Reef, breaks a small smile. "A wilderness program is just life," he says. "But more of it." As the miles unfurl he offers snapshots of his world view, including the notion that there are things to be learned from the hard times in life, that there are both reason and opportunity in the unique ways these kids relate to their surroundings, even though such ways of relating may be awfully inconvenient to those around them.

That, in turn, leaves me thinking back to the girls of Group 3, and the bulging fanny pack of prescription drugs Jonathan had strapped to his waist every waking hour, sleeping with it, calling in the flock three times a day with a cry of "Meds!"—passing out whatever rations of Prozac and Ritalin, lithium and Wellbutrin the psychiatrists back home had prescribed. "So where do prescription drugs fit in with that philosophy?" I ask him. "Aren't some of these kids on drugs because no one has time to deal with that uniqueness you're talking about—no one has time to teach them what to do with it?"

"Sometimes that's true," he says, pausing to remind me that he's not a medical doctor. "We've got one kid in Group Four right now—his therapist back home prescribed a Ritalin placebo, and the kid is convinced it's helping. That's fantastic—I wish more doctors would give that approach a try. But it's hard to argue with therapists who follow the drug model, because

drugs do take away the symptoms. I've seen a few kids out here
taken off their meds and it can leave them a little crazy—more
angry, more depressed, a lot more likely to act out. It's easy to
see why those drugs are so popular."

Brad tells me that from what he's seen so far, this program
works great for ADD kids, also kids with behavioral problems,
maybe not quite so well for depression. "I've only had three
kids taken out. One was violent. The other two just couldn't
keep safe—they were either threatening suicide, or just not willing to take care of themselves."

Like all the therapists here, in addition to two full days a
week with Group 4, Brad also spends a lot of time with a phone
to his ear, talking with parents. What's more, given how Pam,
the therapist for the girls, had to talk her senior instructor
through a serious low point last week, I'm also wondering how
much goes into helping his staff keep it together.

"First of all," he says, "one of the things I like best about
this job is that I get to work with some incredible people in the
field. It's with the instructors that things really get done. That
said, everyone out here is going to go through rough times.
Those who burn out first and worst are the ones who think
they're here only for the kids, not for themselves. If they can't
get in touch with their own needs, if they deny them or repress
them, keep putting them off, they're screwed. They will burn
out. I've seen it time and again." I think back to our training
group. Off the top of my head I'd say at least half of the people
told me they came because they wanted to help, never uttering
a word about what was in it for them.

———

There's no trace of the six inches of fresh snow that fell on the Henry Mountains five days ago; only the steep, west-facing slopes hold any sign that winter was here at all. As we spin down into the desert, patches of locoweed start to appear, their clustered, ivory blooms scattered across the dry lands like puddles of spilled milk. Desert holly is full on now, as are the first of the evening primroses—exquisite, chalice-shaped blooms hanging from middling-looking vines in places with no names.

Spring in the Utah desert is mostly a roller coaster, full of surprises, sort of like a grizzly bear about to clamp his jaws around your head and then deciding instead to cuddle you and lick your face. You sit there trying to enjoy the wonder of it, but always in the back of your head knowing full well that the slightest thing could set him off again. Even the intrepid Mormons, with their uncanny knack for squeezing life out of inhospitable places, have been at various times brought to their knees in this part of Utah, rocked from one extreme to another—searing drought in one season, flooding in the next. After devastating spring floods in the latter 1800s and again in 1909, the church's leader for the area called the faithful to Loa and in an almost unheard-of move, gave them honorable release from their lives here, praying to a generous Father that he bless the people wherever they go, whatever they do. "Someone has said that one man's heaven is another's horror," wrote a local historian. "So it is with Wayne County. A heaven on earth to some, to others, discouragement, disillusionment, despair, disaster, desolation, and death."

Several field staff have suggested that something very different happens to kids when they're in this desert, compared to when

they're high in the forests of Boulder Mountain. More gets done
in the desert, they say. The changes seem to be faster, deeper.
Most think it has something to do with the fact that there are
so few places to hide, no leaf canopies or thickets or tree trunks
to offer refuge. Land as a mirror held up to a kid's life—at first,
harsh as his worst fears, but over time, at least for some, bright
and fierce and wild as youth itself. A land of pain and clarity.

Going from the girls of Group 3 to the boys of Group 4,
I'm about to discover, is sort of like driving out of a thick fog
into the path of a tornado. The fact that I'm jumping between
girls and boys at all is due to a recent move away from coed
groups—a change driven in part by the desire to end the kids'
constant attempts at sex, with the side benefit of giving the girls
a shot at the kind of growth most research says is more likely
to happen in an all-female setting. Some of the staff think it's a
mistake. They regret losing the chance for teenagers to get a
handle on how the other gender sees the world. Still, most agree
that the girls do seem more inclined to be themselves with other
girls, whether that means burping and farting around the campfire, or something a bit more significant, like doing things for
themselves instead of giving in to the guys who are usually stumbling all over themselves to do it for them.

That said, being with the guys over the next eight days,
seeing them willing at the drop of a hat to rocket off to planet
testosterone, I'll end up thinking a little estrogen might be a
good thing. In truth this is the first time in three weeks that
Group 4 will have even a female staff with them. The lucky
winner of that position is Kate, the woman I trained with, the
artist from the apple orchards of Vermont.

The last of our two-hour drive from Bicknell is on five miles
of rutted dirt, followed by the crossing of a sizable creek—

thankfully, not one big enough to get stuck in with two-wheel drive. Brad parks, I grab my backpack, and we begin walking upstream looking for the group. "Just finding the kids can be a challenge sometimes," he says. "Especially for the newer staff, who don't have a working knowledge of the roads and the cow paths." The therapist hired most recently, a large, beaming man named Paul, has been lost every week for the past month.

We find the guys lying around in a grove of cottonwoods, working on journals and growth books and curriculum. Larry, a short, stocky kid wearing thick glasses and a head of hair covered with dust, a nerdy kid turned gnarly, is showing a couple of other boys how to make natural cordage out of yucca leaves. I ask if I can join them, grab some yucca, give it a try.

"I was such a jerk when I came here," Larry says after a while, talking like a guy who needs to get his past off his chest. When I tell him I suppose all of us have been jerks now and then he nods, smiles, and assures me that he was a bigger jerk than most. "I mean what would you say about a kid who's been here for two weeks, slips out of the tent on a winter day, in a sleet storm, lays down outside in his underwear, trying to kill himself?" Even after being rescued by staff Larry continued to playact the hypothermia thing for all it was worth, pretending to be semiconscious so they'd eventually call in air support and get him out. Out for good. He blew it when someone leaned on his chest and he flinched, and then again when one of the staff told her coworker to give him three swallows of water, and after three swallows, having obviously heard what she said, he stopped and pulled his head away.

I'll grant Larry this much: He was one hell of a slow learner. Between his constant lying and his almost hopeless incompetence, he ruffled the feathers of new and seasoned instructors alike. "He was the lowest-functioning student I've ever seen," says Jesse, one of the veteran staff here this week. "He couldn't take care of himself at all. Two weeks here and he still couldn't pack his survival pack—would always have stuff falling out all over the place." Another instructor, this one fresh out of training, spent one week with Larry and remembers him the same way. When later this month I tell him about Larry's incredible ability with hard skills he'll get positively wide-eyed, shake his head as if I'd brought news of a miracle. "He was so full of BS," he'll say. "So unwilling to do anything in his own behalf. I tried for an hour and a half to teach him how to build a bow-drill fire. He finally broke down in tears, and I was damn close to it myself."

At just over a month Larry started coming around, feeling more confident. On Brad's suggestion his parents agreed to keep him in longer—ten weeks instead of eight—and he's only gotten better. Nobody can make cordage or start a bow-drill fire or put up a tarp or carve a spoon like this guy. He's reliable, he's a patient teacher, and the word is he'll make eagle before the week is out. "This program works great," Larry tells me. "But only if you want to change." He says he's not entirely sure himself what prompted the shift. "It had to do with accepting the fact that I was here. I finally quit fighting, just decided to make the best of it, learn what there was to learn."

For the time being, though, the lone eagle is Wade—a cool, tanned seventeen-year-old with freckles and a space between his teeth through which he manages to hurl beads of spit with both impressive speed and frequency. Every couple of minutes he gives his head a good shake, a habit I'm guessing started as a means of tossing his blond hair out of the way, even though these days it's forever pinned tight under the fabric of a red stocking cap. Like other kids he's torn the arms off his gray sweatshirt, but unlike others, his pants are ripped up and down the inside of the thighs to the point where it's easy to see the designs on his cotton boxers. Air-conditioning, he tells me, tossing his head again.

I get the feeling right off that Wade's a smartass, inflated with the power that comes from being senior hood in the woods, confident that as a newcomer I would eventually have to come to him to find out the skinny of what's happening in Group 4. The kind of kid who'll play it cool, probe you with questions of his own until he senses what kind of role he should play with you. Still, he has his qualities. Every now and then I get the sense he's really trying to figure out what leadership is all about. I hear him defend the group, give advice (some of it pretty bad), do favors—not necessarily out of any altruism, more to see if such behavior feels right for his station.

After years of being considered a screw-off in boarding school, Wade definitely has moments when he seems grateful for this new chance, proud of it. And something else, too. After an hour of talking he takes a deep breath, looks around him, drinks in the smell and the sky and the color of the canyon walls. "I didn't know anything about wilderness before I came here. But I love it so much. I'm coming back here, man. I'm coming back."

Next week is Wade's last, and while he hated this place with a passion seven weeks ago, he's not exactly jumping up and down about leaving. "It's sort of bittersweet. I mean it'll be good to get back to my other life, see my girlfriend. But I've had some great times here. The group is going to change with me gone. Now the younger ones will get the feeling of being the experienced ones. That's good. It's time for things to change."

In time a couple of other kids wander over, Ray and Frank, sit down in the sand with us. Ray is a hard-talking, muscular kid—the boy whose parents sat in their living room back in Chicago several weeks after the escorts came, one minute wringing their hands over what their son had become, the next choking on guilt for having sent him here. "We're a bunch of drug users and thieves," Ray tells me, flashing a movie-star smile. "Better watch your stuff around this camp."

Frank on the other hand is a thin, graceful sixteen-year-old, calm almost to the point of being holy. He talks more like a fifties beatnik than a fifties beatnik, not only regularly launching into all manner of commentary about existentialism, but quoting line after line of Kerouac and Ginsberg and Ferlinghetti. Together these two have an incredible amount of personality and brain power; even Wade seems taken aback by them. Brad is off doing one-on-one with the rest of the boys, so for the next hour the four of us lie around on the ground and talk. Ray tells me how, when this is all over, when they finally get their freedom, he and Frank are going to head for Mexico and try to meet up with Carlos Castaneda's Yaqui Indians. "You don't find them," he explains, suddenly looking very serious. "They find you."

When I tell them I'm a writer, Frank and Ray jump up and run off back to their packs, come back a minute later holding smudged sheets of paper with about a half dozen poems, ask if I'd like to hear some. "I write a lot of stuff out on solo," Frank says. "But I trade it. Wipe my bum with it and burn it. Go on, man," he says, nodding to Ray. "Read us somethin'." So Ray shuffles the dirty pages, pulls out one called "I'm Not Crazy."

Who you callin' crazy
You wacko doctor you.
You give me all these pills to pop,
And tell me what to do.
You scan my brain,
You probe my mind,
I call you Doctor Frankenstein.

Who you callin' crazy
Mr. Legal dope dealer
You walk through Savon Pharmacy
Just like a shopping spree.
You say you know what's best,
You say you know what's right,
Someone needs to give you drugs
to make you see the light.

Give me pharmaceuticals
Give me medication
Give me all the drugs you got
Call me a mental patient.
Put me in a padded room
Tie me down with straps
I'd rather be a prisoner
Than with you crazy quacks.

Pump me full of drugs
Make my mind real hazy,
But you'll never take from me the truth—
I'm not the one who's crazy.

It's the first of dozens of angry poems I'll hear from Group 4 in the weeks to come. Curiously, poetry has emerged as the method of choice for these guys to deal with all kinds of emotions, including rage—a turn of events that some staff think is yet another fruit of lots of time spent in this desert. Sam, a stocky, freckle-faced kid from Newark who was sent here in large part because of uncontrollable anger, wasn't here a week before he got ticked off at something, grabbed a stick, and came at an instructor, said he was going to shove it someplace where sticks aren't supposed to go. But this afternoon, and all through the next eight days, I'll see him handle all kinds of frustrating situations, staying fairly mellow the whole time. "The poetry lets me get the anger out," he'll tell me. "I never liked writing at all, but getting it down on paper helps keep it from building up inside. You know, I've written poems to my girlfriend almost every day since I've been here." In truth, most of those have enough detail of certain sex acts to serve as a training manual; even so, there's some real emotion there, too—a sense of relationship.

The same with Jim, who the day before he came here told his parents that if they tried to send him away he'd beat them to death with a flashlight. The journaling he's been doing is full of emotion—lots of stuff about how much he still hurts over having lost his girlfriend last year, how sad he is about his brother leaving home and blowing off the rest of the family. It's a crude thought, but after talking with Sam and Jim I find myself flashing on a tongue-in-cheek comment a wildlife veterinarian friend of mine made when he heard I was coming here. "Don't forget," he said. "The reason Dobermans can be made to be so mean is because they're so incredibly sensitive."

Brad wraps up the one-on-one sessions around two o'clock. Afterward everyone gathers to talk about the group's current problem child, a slight, fourteen-year-old kid named Ruben. Brad sits cross-legged on the ground, baseball hat turned backward, looking down, absentmindedly drawing circles in the sand with his index finger. Finally, after a long silence, he tells the guys he's confused about his meeting with Ruben, doesn't know what he should do, wants their advice. Ruben, meanwhile, looks up only to cast a grin at the others, hoping, no doubt, for the same in return, this time getting nothing. "Ruben told me today that he thinks drugs are good," Brad says, "and that he's way too smart to ever be controlled by them or get caught. He also said going to prison would be fine—a lot better than this." Brad asks if anyone else in the group has anything to say that might help, that he wants to "raise Ruben's bottom" but he's out of ideas. Feeling hopeless.

"Look, Ruben," says Jerry, sweeping long red hair out of his face. "When I was your age I was the same way. I'd heard all the talk, had all the speeches. But I thought the same things you do—that I was too smart to get caught, that I could give it up when I wanted to, all that stuff. I thought the junkies living in the streets in their tattered clothes were cool; I didn't mind being like them at all. Until you hit bottom, man, there's nothing I can do or say."

"It was the same for me, little man," says Ray. "I had to get scared, and then I started changing. Look at you over there, grinning and crap. You're not scared, little man. You're not scared."

Ruben not only hasn't hit his bottom, but like a lot of fourteen-year-olds who come into this program, he's not mature enough to look around the corner, to link what he's done in the past to where he is now. It's hard for him to see how certain decisions he's made about his family—his father abandoning him, his mother's drinking—might have anything to do with how he relates to the world at large. His thinking is concrete; metaphors about personal power, which abound not only in the myths and stories used here, but are a major part of the struggle to live well in the wilderness, tend to bounce right off him.

Many staff, even some therapists, say they'd rather not have

fourteen-year-olds even admitted unless there are strong indica-
tions that the kid is fairly mature—someone like Carla in Group 3,
the girl who thought the cows were going to get her out on
solo. In truth this program is licensed for twelve-year-olds, but
so far the powers that be have had the good sense not to take
them.

Brad tells us that Ruben is to go on separates for the next
several days, which basically means being alone, no interaction
with the group. It's not meant as a punishment for his comments
about drugs, but a consequence of him continually screwing off
in group, smirking at the whole idea of somebody trying to
come to terms with their stuff. The exception to separates, Brad
says, is that anyone who wants to, with a staff person present,
can tell him their stories—their tales of hitting bottom. That
doesn't mean war stories, he reminds them, which is a telling
of past drug larks or criminal frolics in a way that paints them
as romantic or heroic. It's okay to talk about waking up in the
alley behind the Circle K in a puddle of vomit if your point is
how that was the moment when you knew you needed help;
it's not okay to present that image as the funniest night of your
summer vacation.

Besides Kate and me, the staff this week includes a rather celebrated duo, Shawn and Jesse. Shawn, who likes to build his
vacations around multiple Phish concerts, came here as a student five years ago, when he was a senior in high school (or
would have been, had he not gotten kicked out). Interestingly,
he got here pretty much through his own desire, struggling to
change a life that was spinning out of control in a flurry of acting
out and stealing, the final insult when he swiped two thousand

dollars from his mother. He says the biggest thing he got from this place was motivation—that the program left him with the realization that he could take care of himself, which at the time was nothing short of a revelation. "I used to hate pushing those damn carts," he tells me. "Then my instructor, she told me to think of the cart as the one thing in my life that I didn't want to face, that I didn't want to deal with. And that comment turned it all around."

Jesse, on the other hand, is compassionate, an amazingly good listener—the kind of big brother most kids would pick out for themselves if they could assemble a family by ordering it out of a catalog. Together Shawn and Jesse are incredibly funny, guys who could make decent coin working drive-time talk radio instead of trudging through the desert playing policeman and confessor for eight bucks an hour. When the mood is right—which basically means when the boys are trying—break times with these two seem less like adventure programming than Monty Python on wilderness vacation.

It's a four-mile push to the base of Trapper Ridge, through a long, lonesome valley running along the massive headwalls of Capitol Reef, finishing with a brutal climb into the highlands beneath the ridge itself. After tarps are up Kate suggests we hike up to the high ledges and do some drawing. For the next hour I watch the guys out there, intent with their chalk and colored markers, their drawing paper weighted with stones against the wind, sprawled on the lip of this high ridge like so many body surfers riding the crest of a five-hundred-foot wave of stone. The view in three of four directions is outrageous—in the distance great, yawning sweeps of stone; close by, the occasional raven spinning overhead on black, black wings, lizards doing push-ups in the sand.

I'm baffled by how into drawing and painting these kids are, especially given that most say they never had any interest in art. At first I think the effort might be just to please Kate, who receives a surprising amount of respect from them, whose mere presence seems to bring them down slightly from their frenzied orbits. But Jesse thinks it goes deeper than that. Art, he says, like writing or even drumming, is part of something that sprouts all the time out here—a willingness to look inside, grab hold of any thread that seems likely to lead them to their passion.

The end result is a strange mix of macho and inward reach, a bunch of kids perfectly willing to rag on one another for being ugly or stupid or fat, but offering nothing short of mutual reverence for a piece of art or a few lines of poetry, no matter how bad it might be. Whether any of this lasts in the long run, of course, it's impossible to say. But at an age of self-consciousness and cool it seems notable that they're willing to make the journey at all.

It's after dark when we finally settle into dinner—a hodge-podge of bacon and salt pork and ramen and macaroni and cheese eaten with wooden spoons carved from sticks, all set to conversation both sublime and bizarre, sort of a *My Dinner with André* meets *The Wild Bunch*. Frank ends up spinning tales of political intrigue—first about how Ho Chi Minh and his followers used to hold meetings in caves deep in the woods of North Vietnam, followed by a detailed description of a Russian psychopolitical scheme to sanction drugs, sex, and rock and roll as a means of maintaining control over young people. From there we make a quick segue into a series of questions for Dave, the intern instructor, about why he's vegetarian, and just as fast— and this with staff just out of earshot—skate into a war story about a kid Frank knew in boarding school who, in order to conserve his limited supply of drugs, would pick his nose every night, then cut out the chunks of crystal meth so he could bump them again before bed.

Ruben and Ray and I are off by ourselves, sitting in the sun on a slab of sandstone. Ray's decided to take Brad up on his suggestion to work with Ruben one-on-one, try to use his own dance with drugs as a means of helping Ruben get a grip on the stakes of the game. As a frame for the conversation they use a growth book designed to help kids start taking a look at the effects of the decisions they've made. One of the pages asks them to list the costs of their drug habit; Ruben snorts, tells Ray there's hardly been any cost at all.

"C'mon, man," Ray says, shaking his head. "What about your memory? Have you lost any of that?"

"Yeah, well, I guess so. Sometimes I can't remember questions the teacher asked like five minutes before."

"There you go. I can't remember things at all anymore. I don't know if it's from the drugs, or from all the concussions I got when I was high—banging my head into walls."

From there Ray walks Ruben through an accounting exercise of sorts, using a worksheet to make weekly tallies of his drug purchases. Like most kids, when he first got here Ruben lied to beat the band when it came to what kinds of drugs he'd been using, and how often, as though admitting the full story would be a fast track to landing in even more trouble. It all comes out with Ray, though. When the math is finally done and Ray announces the cost of the highs, it causes the first truly surprised look I've seen from Ruben. His two-year cocktail of

PCP, heroine, inhalants, booze, and pot comes to just under nine thousand dollars.

"Man," Ruben says, shaking his head. "For that much I could've had a car."

By the time we load up and start walking again, it's hot, somewhere close to ninety. Two hours out of camp, heading north, we enter the bleakest stretch of desert yet—mile after lonely mile of greasewood and rabbit brush framed by a rumpled blanket of bentonite hills, each bruised with grays and purples, not one of them with a single bush or flower or blade of grass. Walking in the back of the group—just behind Ruben, who's still on separates—on several occasions I've looked up and been startled by the sight, this line of young nomads strung out over a quarter mile along a steep grade, sweating and panting behind their carts. Like a scene from some epic movie, biblical, though this is one covey of pilgrims that has no sense at all of being chosen people. The strangeness continues to grow after we leave the hills and take a break near an old cattle trough, next to a beat-out, 1930-something truck with a monster well-drilling rig on its bed, up to its axles in dried mud, busted and abandoned by its owner to become a pack-rat hotel.

The kids get a big kick out of poring over the machinery, fondling the old wooden flywheels and cracked rubber belts, the funnel-shaped headlights and the mammoth gears layered with rust. Frank especially is fascinated by the thing, starts asking me all sorts of questions about Steinbeck's *The Grapes of Wrath*—what happened to most of the people who headed west to California, and how did their experiences add fuel to the labor movement. His brain moves like lightning, and before long he's leaning against the metal door of the truck, a piece of grass between his teeth, looking so much like Jack Kerouac it's spooky, struggling to draw comparisons between persecution of the Wobblies and the McCarthy hearings of the fifties, and then tying all that into the Vietnam War.

After spinning my head for another fifteen minutes, he settles down, and we walk over to the cattle trough to fill up our water bottle with what amounts to pond scum: It's little wonder most of us have gas that could peel the chrome off a bumper. "My God," Florida Dave is saying. "There are people in Africa who wash their children in wine because the water is so bad. This is just like that." We sterilize the stuff by dropping iodine tablets into the bottles, move over to the shade of an old cottonwood where Frank starts up another conversation, this time telling me how he got here.

"There was this big dude, man, comes into my dorm room at four in the morning and shakes me awake, tells me we're going to Utah. I was still asleep—ended up grabbing my roommate's clothes and his sandals by mistake, which were way too big for me—just walked out like that. It was crazy." Three hours later he was in the Chicago airport, the big escort still at his side, about to board the plane, when he decides to make a break for it, hurling himself out the security door, down the steps and across the tarmac, running like a wild man. "I remember the shoes—my roommate's sandals—I kept tripping over them. Finally kicked them off so I could run better. It was really nuts, trying to stay away from all the vehicles that were buzzing around out there; all the time I kept worrying that I'd end up on a runway where a plane was landing."

With anyone else this would be a war story of the first magnitude. But Frank tells it only as a matter of fact, a straightforward recounting of something he thought he needed to do at the time, no more bluster to the telling than had he been recounting a trip to the store to buy a gallon of milk. After about five or ten minutes running around out there, he explains, he found his way back into the airport, and the security police nabbed him a few minutes later.

Before we head out again, Kate announces she's calling a group—an option open to anyone, anytime. Showing her kindness, she starts out praising the guys, saying how well they seem to be able to work together when they want to, how much she's appreciated them trying new things—playing with the drawing exercises, working with her this morning to make and sculpt clay. "But there's something really bothering me," she says. "Something I need to talk to you about. It's about all the sexual comments. The innuendos you guys make about women, about making it with women. Don't get me wrong. Sex can be a great, fun part of a relationship. But I think you'd find that not just me, but a lot of females would think some of your comments pretty objectionable. All I'm asking is that you try to be a little more conscious about the way you're relating to one another."

Most of the guys look downright chastened, like they've disappointed someone they really care about.

"Sorry, Kate," Jerry says quietly, his head down, and then more "sorries" from Wade and Ray and Frank.

For better or worse, Florida Dave sees an opening here for something that's been on his mind—namely, the insults and verbal abuse the guys level at one another every day. In particular their fondness for making fun of Kevin, the big, disheveled kid I picked up at the airport three weeks ago.

"All you're doing," he says, "is stealing somebody else's energy." He gets looks of boredom and confusion, but no apologies.

The rest of the afternoon centers on Florida Dave, who's

evidently decided that the best way to keep the group on the trailing cart from squabbling is to put out every spark of disagreement he hears, and there're a lot of them. Though you'd never guess it from how wide-eyed and full of squeaky-clean optimism Dave is, in his teen years he was a pretty serious drug user himself. True to the clichés about the fervor of the reformed, he seems determined to enlighten these guys. And if that means kneeling on their chests and force-feeding them some wisdom, then so be it.

We all see it. He's trying too damn hard. When the kids talk about some beer commercial they think is cool, Dave condemns drinking. When he overhears Ray tell someone he still wants to do drugs, he pounces, demanding to know what that will mean for his life, missing the last half of Ray's comment—namely, that he can't do them because he can't control the habit.

Ruben is Dave's special nemesis, sneering at damn near everything Dave says to him, mouthing curses behind his back, prompting Dave to turn up the heat even more. Dave tells me that Ruben reminds him of himself at fourteen, and he seems something just short of desperate to save Ruben from the same grief he went through. From my place at the back of the parade I can see how the guys are starting to resent him, the smirks and snide remarks beginning to brew. By three o'clock, at the tender age of twenty-two, Dave looks a lot like the parent of a troubled teen, tearing his hair out because, *Damn it, these kids just won't listen!* Walking with him later in the afternoon he seems beaten down, losing hope. "I'm beginning to see just how tough this is," he says sadly. Indeed, that incredible enthusiasm he showed in training, talking about wanting to be here at least a year, working with other people who are struggling for their own positive solutions, has taken a major hit. Now he talks only of trying to make it through the summer.

At one point he and Kate walk together for a couple of miles; Dave wants to know if she has any advice for him. She slows her walk, thinks for a minute. "Maybe when Kevin was saying how the cart was going all over the place, that it was heavy, all he really wanted was somebody to listen. I think what he wants is for us to recognize he's suffering. But that's not something he's ever going to come right out and ask for."

It helps. By late afternoon he's started to back off a bit, willing to listen to the chaos without trying to fix it. Tomorrow, before heading out of the field, Dave will ask for a feedback group with the kids, a chance for them to let him know what they think. "Have fun, man," Ray will tell him. "Don't be so heavy all the time." Lead instructors Shawn and Jesse will talk to Dave as well, off to the side, reminding him that these guys are brilliant at spotting somebody who's not coming from the heart. If you're speaking from your head all the time, they'll tell him, spouting clichés, as far as these kids are concerned you're talking from your ass.

The thick light of late afternoon is falling on a desert that seems to be utterly jumping out of its skin with spring. We roll past primrose and cliff rose, wild onions and pepperbrush, globe mallow and holly, and long, soft blankets of phlox. Hanging from every wind is the tangy smell of piñon and juniper—gifts of the so-called pygmy forest, which sprawls across some forty thousand miles of the Southwest, all the way into Old Mexico. We park it late in the evening at Horsetail Seep, which is cradled by thick walls of sculpted sandstone and a quiet pool of sour water where the bats come out to dine on the wing, flashing through grainy clouds of gnats in the last of the light.

Tonight's fireside poetry slam—or the Group 4 Poetry Corner, as some are starting to call it—is long and winded and full of angry groping for place and power. Even a fairly new arrival named Curt—a studly, macho marine-in-the-making—decides to give reading a try, though he seems embarrassed enough about it to wait until dark, when no one can see his face. His piece is a violent one, based on a dream where he finds himself "cutting and shooting at some poor fucker trying to get away," apparently taking no small amount of pleasure in it, only to have that image shift in a blink to exactly what his life is all about right now—pushing carts.

Larry's poem, on the other hand, is full of a different kind of power seeking—namely, bashing the locals of Utah, whom he imagines to be a cluster of hooligans, rhyming on about their lack of teeth and about how theirs "is a family tree that has no branches." Such commentary is one of his favorite themes, though only in front of the group. It strikes me as a hint of his vulnerability—a chance to remind everyone that while he may not be able to kick ass literally, with his fists, at least he can get some good licks in with his wit.

Sam goes last, reading a piece he wrote earlier in the afternoon during journal time, called "Stupid Fucking Fly," which is about just that. And while that may not seem like anything of consequence, the fact is it's one of the first pieces of writing (outside the graphic, gritty lovemaking poems he writes to his girlfriend) that shows resignation about something that's pestering him (the fly), instead of simply fantasizing about destroying it.

———

Little Larry, the kid who seven weeks ago tried to kill himself by lying down on the ground in his underwear and freezing to death, is about to become an eagle. Even more amazing is the fact that being an eagle seems to be the thing he wants most in all the world. It happens in late afternoon, by surprise, Wade coming up from behind and blindfolding him, then leading him to a quiet place in the desert well away from camp, with Kate, Jesse, and me trailing behind. Jesse whispers to the rest of us that although he doesn't think Larry's aware of it, and that neither he nor Shawn planned it, this ceremony is about to happen less than a hundred yards from where he was dropped off as a mouse back in early March. "He was crying a lot, and I remember I had to keep telling him to put his hat on, it was so cold. It was the night before staff change, and I kept having this thought—man, here's a kid who just might try suicide."

But today Larry sits on the sand with back straight and head up, looking enthralled even behind the blindfold. The rest of us take turns telling him what being an eagle means to us. Kate squats down, leans close, rests her fingers on his arm. She says being an eagle is about owning your own stuff, about taking responsibility not just for leading the group but for marshaling your own movement. It's about having the courage to go where you know you need to go. Wade says much the same thing, that Larry has to be plugged in to the group without getting caught up in the group's crap.

Jesse seems nearly as moved as Larry is. "Sometimes during a hectic week it's hard to get up for a transition ceremony," he'll tell me later. But not this time. "This one symbolized a real accomplishment—that kid did what nobody, least of all himself, thought he would ever do." Toward the end of the ceremony

Jesse pulls a poem from his pocket, something he wrote just for
Larry, a gift to take with him when he leaves.

> Out here is where the magic happens,
> here in the quiet, gentle hills.
> Here is where you have cried out
> with moans as deep as the earth.
> Here is where you have found your long-lost
> precious self that the madness took away.
> You will leave part of yourself here,
> but you will take all the hope in the world with you.
> So when you get back to those people
> who talk big in large rooms, you will know this:
> You have been silent in places too beautiful for words.

We finish the ceremony by handing Larry his eagle bead
and an honest-to-goodness backpack, and rise to find the beginnings of an incredible sunset. Half the sky is filled with alternating bands of rose and gold and powder blue, while the
other half—the part hanging over the Henry Mountains—is
washed in the deepest, richest shades of lavender imaginable.
The entire group stops in mid-squabble when they see it, and
every kid walks out onto the elevated ridges of stone lying beyond camp, just stands there, watching. Many native cultures
claim there's no such thing as coincidence on the day of a rite
of passage, and I can't help but wonder if Larry is thinking of
this show as meant for him—the final movement of a passage,
one last great sky before he goes. "Man, I'm really gonna miss
this place," he says to no one in particular. Later, just before
dark Jesse goes off with him, leading him up the canyon so he
can lie down in the exact spot he first laid down in as a mouse,
seventy-four days ago. When they return, Larry is wiping away
a stream of tears.

It's typical on the ride out of the field for staff to give each other feedback, process whatever was going on so there's a better chance of everyone not obsessing about it during their six days off. Florida Dave is still shaking his head over how many mistakes he made, though he seems a little less fatalistic about his chances to get it right in the weeks to come. "If all I manage to be is this chattering box of pseudowisdom," he says, "the kids are going to shut down. I guess I'm starting to see that I'm just a piece of the process—not the whole thing." For the rest of the ride he's quiet, staring out the window into the long runs of desert—realizing, maybe, that right now he needs this place as much as anyone.

Though I've only been in eight days, the ride out seems alarming; forty miles an hour feels like seventy. And then the houses, with their electric lights and trimmed yards, their refrigerators and microwaves and televisions. Pickups cruising by with the radio turned up. Big dogs straining against big chains, barking and whining into a hard wind.

Two and a half hours later we're out, though not necessarily disengaged. Jesse is headed to Bicknell to the only liquor store within sixty miles—the clinic, as he likes to call it—to buy a couple of beers, then to the Aquarius to rent a mindless movie or two. Dave goes home and picks up his guitar, spends a couple of hours playing some old favorites. Kate leaves for Torrey, for home, to do some sketching. I try to write, end up bored and full of fidget— ADD by association, maybe—head down to the Aquarius to drink coffee. I leave the restaurant in the last of the light, walk back home, toss my pack into the van, and hit the road.

CHAPTER SEVEN

CRUISING

MY SO-CALLED DAYS off, the first in more than a month. What a joke. Running up and down Highway 12 like a wolf in a pen. Climbing into ponderosa and sweeps of aspen thick with catkins, then down again through the layers of stone—Wingate and Chinle and Moenkopi—from the Fremont to the Escalante, Oak Creek to Calf Creek, all the way around to Fish Lake. Just getting oriented, I tell myself—casting for a better sense of the land. But the wandering probably has less to do with figuring literal landmarks than figurative ones, trying to place Ruben's hunger for drugs or Curt's willingness to be a cold "father's little marine," Nancy's throwing up, and Susan's wanting to die. And all of that stuck between RVs full of Germans bound for Bryce

Canyon, and plump men from New Jersey with thin white legs
crawling out of Chryslers to snap pictures of Chimney Rock and
the Castle, some looking bored, squinting into the desert like it
was a weight.

The normal work schedule is eight days with the kids, then
six days off. Utterly reasonable. Still, for a lot of instructors taking time off is the hardest part of the job. Some have the good
sense to get out of town. Most of the rest spend half their time
huddled around cups of coffee in somebody's kitchen or at the
Aquarius, passing around memories from the past week in the
field like plates of leftovers, everyone gorging until somebody
finally grows sick of it and suggests a bike ride, or a climb up
the Horn, or for those who tend more toward the sedate, a
movie on the VCR, with—assuming they're not twelve-stepping
themselves—a cold bottle of Optimator or Samuel Smith Oatmeal Stout within easy reach.

It isn't that there haven't been some exciting things, exciting people in this part of the country. Ed Abbey, for one, back and
forth so many times even he lost count. Wallace Stegner, too, feet
up at his cabin on the Fish Lake Plateau, massaging the chill out of
late summer nights with a piñon fire in the stove, by day making
slow, careful forays through the tiny towns of Koosharem, Burr-
ville, and Coyote. But when it's all said and done, Wayne County
is mostly about nice Mormon people who drink neither coffee
nor beer, who don't tend to go out dancing (with the exception
of the high school junior prom, which is attended by absolutely
everyone, from sister and brother to Mom and Dad to Grandma
and Grandpa). For the most part you just don't run across early
twenty- and thirty-somethings whose fun tickets aren't already
pretty well punched by marriage, full-time jobs, and a couple of
kids with another on the way. As a field instructor, whatever

sense of community you end up pasting together around here is going to be made up largely of other people who work for the wilderness program. Which is why all too often the typical conversation ends up going something like this:

"So how was Tricia doing?"

"Better, but her father wrote her this really crappy letter, said she wasn't pulling her weight, that she never had—all this really harsh stuff."

"You're kidding! What's up with that guy? I heard he dropped out of therapy last week—said his wife and the therapist were ganging up on him."

"I really hope she gets to go on to another program. Going home would be a killer—"

"Hey, man, wait a minute. We're doing it again. No more shop talk, damn it! How about a beer?" Gets up, grabs two bottles of Slickrock Ale from the fridge, returns, sits down on the couch, hands one of the beers to his companion.

"Yeah, I really think if Tricia can get past the anger thing, she's going to be all right," the companion says. "There's all that stuff with her mother. This week she started talking about it—she's definitely dealing with it, not just with staff, but in group."

"Excellent. God, she's such a great kid. So what about Nancy? What a tough case she is . . ."

And on it goes like this, sometimes for hours, sometimes for days. When the weather turns bad your thoughts drift out into the desert or onto the Boulder and you fret, wondering if everyone's all right. If you're not careful the dreams begin, program dreams, and before long they're coming nearly every night. Keep going down that road, and you may start feeling a loss of enthusiasm, then depression. It's little wonder that anybody

who's been here six months without taking enough extra time
off to fill up the tank and drive across the Utah state line is
considered either a prodigy or a fool. Some arrange for regular
counseling sessions with therapists in surrounding towns. Steve
says he buys beer and watches television, that all he wants to
do is be a vegetable. "I see these bumper stickers on cars saying
SHOOT YOUR TV," he snorts. "Shoot your own fucking TV!" The
day after that comment he revealed a plan for this coming Feb-
ruary—still work as staff, but stay in the backcountry on his days
off. Spend four or five months out in the wild, pay twenty-five
bucks to someone on the other shift to bring him boxes of food,
cigarettes, the occasional bottle of Jim Beam. I'm thinking
maybe this is what burnout looks like for Steve.

I stop along the highway twice today to make bow-drill
fires, though for the life of me I can't say why. By early evening
I'm back at the Aquarius, drinking coffee, chatting with Steve
and Shawn and Tim, an old friend of Shawn's from Nashville who
came out to work just over a year ago. Unlike Shawn, Tim isn't a
former student here, but he definitely knows the words to all the
music, having himself been tossed out of high school into a thirty-
day lockdown rehab facility, where he began what would become a three-year daily practice of Alcoholics Anonymous.

Steve and Shawn are discussing relationships, how tough
it is in this job to have any kind of significant other. "Man,"
Shawn says, "I can't see myself ever getting into it with someone
until I quit this. After eight days out there I'm so spent I can't
imagine dealing with the emotional stuff that's part of a relationship. Honestly, I'd go nuts."

Steve agrees. "Maybe if you got with somebody else who
worked here. Sometimes that seems okay. At least they'd understand your exhaustion."

"I don't know. I just got a place up in Salt Lake City—
sharing it with two construction workers who have absolutely
nothing to do with this place. Hey, probably my closest friends
are working here. But with nonprogram people I can disconnect
from what goes on instead of always living this life—the stories,
the rehashing it all over and over again."

Eventually Steve and Shawn head out. Tim and I stay behind, staring out the window into the empty streets of Bicknell,
making small talk with our waitress, Debbie; watching the rail-
road clock on the wall go off every hour, whistling, hissing
steam, sending a plastic train rolling once around the outside of
the face. I don't mean to start going off again, really I don't,
especially when neither of us has been more than a day from
the kids. I can't help wondering, though, how this sort of program compares to Tim's own experience in a rehab center.
Thankfully, he's no more inclined to disconnect than I am, so
we order a couple of plates of fries, take yet another round of
coffee, and he carries on.

He talks about rehab much the way that Susan and Sara
talk about the suicide wards, saying how there was always the
chance to distract himself with TV, pool tables and Ping-Pong
tables, a stocked fridge. He could sleep until two o'clock in the
afternoon if he felt like it. "Don't get me wrong, the therapist
was totally awesome. And there were definitely times when I
broke down in tears—missing my family, coming to realize
things about myself. We all wanted to become better people. It
just wasn't a challenging environment. We weren't stressing out
at the thought of having to push a heavy cart up this steep hill
first thing in the morning because we didn't make it last night.
There wasn't Johnny, who I'm having a problem with twenty-

four hours a day, and I have to figure out some way to deal with him."

Tim says nearly everyone he knows who went through treatment got something out of it. Some got a lot. "But you have to keep in mind that most of it's very indoctrinating. Boom, boom, boom—this is what AA's about, and this is what's going on with you. Out here we're set up to let a kid fly or flounder on his own—give him some situations, but then as much as possible let him figure it out for himself. It's totally different. Ninety percent of the kids who come here have drug or alcohol issues. We use the twelve-step stuff, and a lot of them need to be in AA or NA when they get out if they're going to have a ghost of a chance of making it. But while they're here, there are other options."

If you know how to back off and let the place work for the kid, Tim tells me, the learning can be incredible. For example, he says that few of the staff he works with come right out and tell a kid drugs and alcohol are horrible and they should quit them. It's more about trying to get someone to take a look at where his or her life is, maybe figure out what mistakes they've made, think about where things are going. Then help them see how drugs fit into that. "It's the wilderness setting that makes that kind of inner work happen. Especially when you're deep into it, like on solo. Look, if I'm out on solo and I'm bored to tears, look who it is I'm bored with. If I need to do drugs or whatever around home twenty-four hours a day so that I'm not around myself, maybe that's something to take a look at. What is it I'm so uncomfortable with?

"Every now and then you see a kid come back from a solo, and there's such a difference. She's had this spiritual awakening.

That's why you hear so many staff talking about going on their own solos—we see what it does for the kids."

By the next day I've settled down a bit, manage some reading, listen to some music. After dinner our hulking nineteen-year-old landlord, Jade, comes around, wanting to talk. When he hears I'm from Montana it sparks a fullblown recounting of a trip he and his brother made to the Pryor Mountain Wild Horse Range last summer, where they rode like bats out of hell on the tails of the stallions. After sharing such a story I guess he figures we're pretty good friends, because the next thing I know he wants very much to take me out into the rain to show me his 1984 Chevy shortbed, with dual exhausts and neon glow lights under the rocker panels, hand polished with sixty-dollar-a-bottle wax, so shiny you can see the reflection of the vacancy sign from the Sunglow Motel shimmering in the chrome wheels. "Man, look at the way that rain beads up!" And of course a stereo with enough sound to fill a high school gym, though one speaker isn't working quite right anymore.

"Hey, let's go for a ride," he says.

So this is how I end up spending my time off. Running up and down the main street of Bicknell with country music blaring through a fuzzy speaker and Jade marveling at the rain beading on the hood and windshield of the pickup. It's Friday, cruising night. A half dozen other guys, all solo, spot Jade's truck and wave. How weird—all these guys driving around by themselves, no females in sight, each one trying to impress the other but of course nobody really buying into it. We park in the lot of the Aquarius for a while, run into a couple of friends of Jade's, Mike and John, heading into the restaurant to ask one of their moms—a waitress—if they can stay the night at the other's house. When John first sees me sitting in the passenger seat he flashes a look of panic. "Fuck, man," he says. "I thought you were the sheriff!"

The problem is that once I fall into this cruising thing, I can't seem to get out. The term "merry-go-round" starts taking on a whole new meaning. Around 11:30 we end up in the parking lot of the Sunglow Motel, beside another truck, this one belonging to Andrew. He and Jade spend the next twenty minutes reliving their last great moment of high school, a senior bus trip to Nevada that, while supposedly chaperoned, sounds less like a class outing than an Everclear festival. When Andrew hears I've been working up at the wilderness program he gets a grin on his face, tells me about being up at Donkey Reservoir last fall, tracking a deer, when he hears this noise coming from the bushes. "I pull back the brush, there's a couple of kids from that program doing the nasty. Man, were they surprised."

Boredom sets in, and when it does, the guys decide it would be great fun to see whose stereo is loudest—Jade blasting out Diamond Rio, while Mike lets loose a raucous, head-pounding run of AC/DC Live. The owners of the Sunglow peer out the back window of the place, looking frustrated but not altogether surprised. I'm all ready to say a fast good-bye and make a run for it. Then again, I don't really want to fling open the door on this boombox and walk across the street into the house I'm renting with half of Main Street looking on. So I scrunch down a little farther in the seat, go with it, break into a smile. Jade sees it, assumes I'm enjoying the music, turns it up even louder. That's okay, I tell myself. It's been nearly an hour, and I haven't thought of Ruben or Nancy or Susan even once.

CHAPTER EIGHT

STUBBORN, THY NAME IS BRENDA

ANOTHER STAFF CHANGE, and it's back to the girls of Group 3. In the lead this time is Jimmie—a graceful, if somewhat urgent man with waist-long dark hair and the smile of a prophet. Behind him are Steve ("Shoot your own . . . TV!"), Elizabeth of Appalachian Trail fame, and finally, yet another of the twenty-somethings I trained with, a woman named Emily—calm, cool-headed, reliable, exactly the kind of person you'd want by your side when the cow chips hit the fan. The morning begins, as every Wednesday does, with staff from every group circled up on the lawn at base, and Tony, the field director, handing off all the news we can use—reviewing logistics, answering questions, passing out activities that might make things a little better out in the trenches. Even sharing an inspiring quote now and then. From there it's off to a huddle in front of a massive topographic map, figuring out exactly who's going where, and when, coordinating with other groups to make sure we're not all trying to occupy the same space at the same time. Then gather food and supplies, pick up the meds, load up the truck, stop at the IGA to buy some goodies for the outgoing staff, and by noon hit the road for what's supposed to be a two-hour tour.

But not this time. Yesterday evening a house-size boulder came crashing down onto the highway in the middle of Capitol Reef, missing a school bus by about five minutes, closing the road for the next several days. We'll have to take the Burr Trail instead, nearly doubling the travel time. To make life even more interesting, an hour out of Loa the Dodge truck craps out, and Jimmie and I end up under the hood with a roll of duct tape, reanchoring the solenoid wire—a repair that will still be in place exactly as we made it when I finally leave Utah, six weeks later. An almost perfect record so far: Every time I climb into one of these vehicles it breaks down. Leaning over the engine I tell Jimmie the parents should feel really good knowing that the seventeen thousand dollars it costs them to have a kid in this program isn't being wasted on cars.

Still, it's a pleasant enough place to play mechanic. Along these high reaches the aspen are going from catkin to leaf, pushing a thin green mist across the gray, otherwise lifeless-looking mountain. Lower down, along the Burr Trail, among the great scoops of Wingate sandstone, are long runs of flowers: primrose all over the place, as well as gilia, penstemon, barrel cactus, and, farther down still, acres and acres of rice grass, covering the desert floor with thick blankets of lavender and rust. I've probably seen a dozen springs in the Southwest. None has come close to this.

Since most of us haven't worked together before, Jimmie makes a point of talking about procedures—suggests we staff up twice a day, reminds us of the importance of backing each other up when it comes to laying out consequences, that sort of thing. During our meeting with the outgoing staff, Danielle mentions that we should keep on top of Tricia and a new girl, a fifteen-year-old with severe ADD named Heather, who together have a special fondness for huddling up to talk trash about people. "Also, Heather's been crying a lot—actually broke her solo two days ago, came running into camp screaming because of a rash she found on the side of her leg." And the other new kid, Brenda. A girl who's "really, really angry." The rest of the staff lines out the consequences currently in place, so we can stay consistent, and then we huddle up with the kids and listen to them recount their week.

It's a long session. Nancy tells about a letter from her parents, in which they basically said she was a bad person. The good news, maybe even great news, is that it's been a full week since she threw up, and that includes three days on solo. Sara, meanwhile—the bipolar queen of smudge—is in tears over what she calls a bogus contract with her mom and dad, in which she's been given a choice of either coming home for a month and then leaving for a boarding school, or going there right from Utah.

By far the biggest shock is Susan, the depressed kid I picked up at the airport—the one who as a mouse could hardly crawl out of her sleeping bag. She looks absolutely great. Strong and fit with a sunburned nose, tossing off more smiles in a single hour than I saw last time in an entire week. She's eager to fill us in on a big-time mountain climb the group did a few days ago, gaining more than three thousand feet to the summit of Mt. Pennel. Two-thirds of the way up some of the girls wanted to turn back, leaving the group no choice but to do a sitdown and try to work it out. The "Let's do it" contingent won out, and Susan was one of its strongest voices. I can hardly believe it. The departing staff says she's hiding out a lot less, not spending so much time trying to keep her moods away from the rest of the group. A month from now, at graduation, she'll explain it as learning to see a parallel between the hard physical work she had to do and the difficult emotional work. "After a while, hiding out just didn't seem worth the effort."

Nearly as surprising is Jenna, just back from a special three-day outing known as a quest, which therapists often initiate for a kid who seems either close to a breakthrough or desperately in need of one. Typically it includes two carefully chosen staff and one student, a modest-to-extraordinary amount of hiking and exploring, and lots of intensive talks. If there's anything in this program that seems close to magic, the quest is it. There should be more of them. To nearly everyone here, staff and students alike, Jenna has always seemed incredibly capable. Finally, she thinks so too. "I'm going for eagle," she tells us, even though two weeks ago she was badmouthing the whole idea, in large part because it brings with it a lot of leadership demands. "I'm not totally comfortable with it. But I think it will help me grow." Unknown to staff, this morning she sat down with Nancy and started drafting a letter to her twenty-six-year-old boyfriend— the guy willing to beat her up at the drop of a hat—calling it quits.

The happening of the afternoon, though, is Jonathan announcing that rather than head out of the field for his six days off, he'll instead walk out of camp onto Spider Mesa for a four-day fast. That causes stares of disbelief in some of the girls, especially Brenda, one of the newcomers, who delivers one of those "Are you completely stupid?" looks that absolutely nobody does better. She's even more amazed when Jonathan asks the group to be part of a send-off ceremony he's orchestrated. He has a final confab with Jimmie, going over instructions one last time, and then all of us circle up on the road in the twilight, with Jonathan sitting just off to the side. When everything's quiet, Jimmie lights a frond of sage, carries it over to Jonathan, and smudges him with the smoke, then asks: "By what right do you enter this circle?"

"By way of two gifts," Jonathan replies. "Perfect love and perfect trust." Jimmie then leads him into the center of the circle, turns him north, toward Jenna. "You are facing north," she says, looking a little embarrassed. "North is the direction of the earth." From there he turns slowly clockwise, facing one by one the girls who have volunteered to stand at the cardinal points of the compass, each recounting a small piece of an ancient interpretation of the four directions he's written down for them: "You are facing east," Carla says with astonishing gravity. "East is the direction of air." On it goes. Tricia next, in the south, looking proud about her announcement that this is the direction of fire; and finally Sara, west, home of water.

The spin complete, Jonathan kneels down, reaches his fingers into a billy pot containing a slurry of water and campfire charcoal, and begins to blacken his face. Jimmie asks the rest of us to look through him as if he were transparent, exactly as Tecumseh's people did at the start of his vision quest, exactly as the people of countless young men through the ages in cultures around the world have done.

Jonathan rises. Jimmie tells him to go, to "leave this sacred place, leave it and find one of your own." And with that he walks off toward the northeast, slowly, eyes to the ground, finally disappearing in a wash cradled with holly flowers and primrose. The girls are shaking their heads, and I can tell they want to talk about it. But they also sense the need to simply carry on—knowing that Jonathan considers that to be part of the ritual, too; and they like Jonathan far too much to do anything that might cheapen his experience. We all head back to camp in silence, start gathering wood, bust out a bow-drill fire, go back to living the mundane life, the life of the ones left behind.

The next day is slow and hot. From the time we break one camp to the time we make the next, we manage no more than a mile, mostly because Pam decides to conduct her therapy sessions in place instead of on the move. She finds us on the trail about noon, does a short check-in with the whole group, then begins individual sessions. Those run for more than three hours, and after that she hikes with us, helps set up camp, carries on with her one-on-ones from there.

Tonight is one of those incredibly sweet evenings when I find myself wishing that the whole lot of us were tribal for good. Huddled together in this desert staring into the flames, clocking the passing of the night by lifting our eyes to watch the drift of the Dippers and the Pleiades. The bagels we made are drying beside the fire, and the air is full of the smell of garlic and dough. Jimmie has his small battered guitar with him, and he and Emily pass it back and forth, Jimmie playing his own concoctions—

something halfway between David Wilcox and Michael Hedges—
while Emily goes with the Indigo Girls. Elizabeth is here, too,
answering lots of questions about her two thousand miles on
the Appalachian Trail.

"I wanna do that!" Nancy and Jenna say.

It's well past ten when Pam surfaces from underneath a
nearby juniper to take a breath, still two girls to go. She's going
to be out of town next week at a conference, and has asked
Jimmie to do parent calls for her. She cautions him gently about
the way he's been encouraging the girls to become advocates
for their own lives once they get out of here—exploring ways
of working with their parents to find some level of compromise.
Personally that approach seems plumb to me. Pam, though,
points out the downside.

"You've got these fourteen- to sixteen-year-olds," she's saying, "and after all these years their parents are finally deciding
to get tough, lay down some rules and stick to them. Parents
who've finally figured out that it was more important to be effective, than be popular." She mentions a time recently when
Jimmie suggested to Sara that maybe she could help decide what
aftercare program she'll go to, says that kind of talk might not
make things any easier. "I'm trying to encourage these moms
and dads to take the reins back from kids who have been holding them for years. We need to support them doing just that."

It's a fine and confusing line—at least for me, maybe for
Jimmie, too. So many of these kids have parents who've
dropped the ball, may always drop the ball, and so you try to
get a kid to take responsibility for his or her own well-being, to
not play the victim role because sooner or later that turns into
a dead end. At the same time, there are parents out there who've
made plenty of bad choices in the past, but now, through a lot

of sincere effort, are coming out with fresh determination to do
things right, to give their kids relationship, structure. Which is
more fruitful out here in the great wide open? Encourage a
fifteen-year-old to give the parents she doesn't trust another
chance—give them a shot at doing their job—or find ways to
help the kid entrench an emerging identity that, while perhaps
fundamentally different from what her parents think is appropriate, could end up defining the lion's share of the character
she'll have to lean on in the years to come?

Jimmie, as much as any staff I've met, is a fervent, passionate advocate for these kids—a man who some see as a kind of
long-suffering hero. Maybe it has something to do with his own
memories of being small, picked on, a survivor of abuse and
divorced parents, a well-meaning mother always telling him:
"It's okay if you're little—I'll always be here to take care of
you."

"I did everything I could to gain an identity," he tells us,
fishing a bagel from the edge of the coals with a gloved hand.
"Drugs, vandalism, whatever." Yet in the telling he never
sounds like a victim—more a historian, if anything, mapping out
the roads that led him to the place he is right now. "I've always
learned more down in the troughs of the waves," he says, "than
I ever have up on the crests." There were two adults who kept
him from self-destructing: a Boy Scout leader, and a youth volunteer at his church. "They were the first people who ever just
talked to me, treated me not like I was a kid but another human
being. It's because of them that I relate to these kids the way I
do, on their level, like they're human."

Jimmie can listen with uncommon intensity, investing himself to the point where I wonder how in the world he manages
to keep it going. Last week he had to leave the field because of

a severe rash spreading fast across much of his body. The driver from backup came to get him right as Jenna was telling him something important, so Jimmie plunked himself down in the sand with her and spent the next hour and a half helping her to work it out—a move that didn't exactly earn him any brownie points with the guy sent to pick him up. Similarly, we got word recently that we'll be going up to the mountain soon, and need to be at Notom Bench by a certain day for pickup. Jimmie balked, saying how given the heat and what was going on in the group, it was too much of a march to manage.

Clearly, part of what keeps him sane is that for the six months of the year he's not in Utah, mentoring kids, he's on a homestead in Alaska, some two hundred miles north of Denali, eight miles from the nearest road, in a log cabin he and some friends built with their own hands, dragging everything in on their backs, including a wood stove and a clawfoot bathtub. He writes and brews beer and sits in that clawfoot tub—which, by the way, is outside, at the edge of the woods—taking long, deep breaths of the wild. "Sometimes people will come up to me and say, 'Hey, your life is going to catch up to you. What sort of plans do you have for the future? What are you going to do when you're fifty?' Every time I'm out in nature I'm struck by the authenticity of it—plants reaching for the light, animals making a living, everything doing the best it can. I'm just trying to do the same."

From the looks of things, Pam is facing the usual range of upheaval tonight. Nancy's moved away from outright fear of her father, wanting only to please him, showing instead some honest-to-goodness anger. She's written a letter to her dad calling him on his habit of throwing his power at everyone around the house, badgering her mother. Dad didn't take that well and is grumbling to the education consultant about Pam not being a very good therapist. He says all the staff here are being snowed, that Nancy's bulimia isn't that serious—more a ploy for attention than anything else. Despite his agreement to do the therapy thing—the agreed-upon counseling sessions for the duration of Nancy's stay—Dad says it "just isn't working out" for him.

Several of the girls are helping me tend the bagels, munching one when possible, eagerly awaiting the next. One of the newcomers, Heather, who's prone to breaking down in tears at the drop of a hat, says she's relieved finally to get some help with the drug thing—that she's tried to quit before and just couldn't. "I've been high for four years," she tells me. "I don't have a clue who I am. I'm sad, but I'm scared to find out." She tells about running away from home and staying a few days in a condo belonging to a friend's parents, then joining up with a couple in their fifties, the woman being an ex–Hell's Angel, but "really, really nice." It was on that door her father finally knocked, having looked for her for nearly a week. I ask what he said.

"He was cool," she says. "He said I could have a couple more days, that I should come home when I'm ready." She finishes with a story about this friend of hers who set fire to some gang member's car, how he was hiding out when she left. Tonight she'll wake up in tears, shaken to the bone by a dream that the gang found and killed him. Heather is the kind of kid who leaves me praying for aftercare.

It never ceases to amaze me how easily the girls can be locked in conversations about the most grueling situations one minute, and the next be begging for bagels, playing the Stick Game, laughing to tears. Everyone except Brenda, that is. She sits on the outside of the circle with a frown on her face, throwing disdainful looks at everyone, staff and students alike.

She's no better the next morning. An hour before we're ready to leave she sits down in the middle of camp and says she's not going anywhere. "Just leave me here to die. Just blow my head off—I'd rather be dead than be here." Over and over again. "Look, you guys can just leave me here, and I'll write a note that I ran away so none of you will get in any trouble. By the time they find me I'll be dead."

Jimmie, who most days has enough patience in his pockets to warm the heart of a terrorist, gets absolutely nowhere with her. Steve goes next, then Elizabeth, and despite their best efforts the ice on the pond just keeps getting thicker. No one's really trying to get her to hike so much as just let her know she can loosen her grip, make some connections with people, get from this side of the program to the other without white knuckles and clenched fists. But her survival strategy is to build walls, big ones, and in the end the rest of the group tosses their packs aside, circles up under a tree and begins curriculum. Thirty yards away I sit with Brenda, just hang out with her, remind her that it's okay if she doesn't want to walk, tell her that I know she's way too smart to think we could really leave her out here in the desert to die.

"You won't get in trouble," she says again, exasperated. "I told you: I'll tell them I ran away when you weren't looking, and you won't get into trouble. Look, I don't care about my life. I'm not worth it," though she says it less like someone depressed than defiant. In truth Brenda is smart, very smart, able to fly through classes in school, pulling down A's without even thinking about it; a lot of what she says feels like a test, round one in a long, dreary game of "shock the staff." Indeed, in the days to come Brenda will pull out all stops in her attempts to horrify us, use every conceivable tack to push our buttons—telling us how stupid she is, sharing her vision of heaven as a place with shelves filled with heroine, where she's the only prostitute. She'll work every staff person a little differently, and seem increasingly astonished when no one bites, when all most of them do is rub their chins and say in a genuinely curious voice, "Really? What would be the advantage of that?"

Her mother has said that while Brenda uses the "I wanna die routine" constantly, she's never shown the slightest interest in suicide. Still, she's alarmed at the throwaway attitude Brenda has about life. In the past six months she's been hanging out with a local gang—the same gang that one of her best friends died in last winter, victim of a brutal knifing.

We end up sitting together for more than three hours. Halfway through she quits jousting with me long enough to give a tiny glimpse into what life was like for her back in Michigan. She tells of a month spent doing inhalants—Glade air freshener, mostly, day after day—how it started out as the most amazing rush but ended with her hating it, worrying about what it had done to her memory. "Even now I can't remember like I could a year ago," she says, careful not to sound sad about it. She talks about the drugs—the pills and the booze and the pot, what she likes about each of them, then is suddenly horrified by a memory of lying in her bed with her clothes on, next to some guy, high on Glade, and without knowing it was coming, peeing all over herself. Had she decided to do that for a lark it would have been one thing. But it was beyond her control; and for Brenda, that's about as far from a lark as you can get.

Around noon she starts talking about her older brothers having taught her "what it is boys are about," leaving me with the notion of a couple of guys sitting down with their little sister to give big-brother warnings about the dangers of testosterone-laden teenage boys, missing altogether what she really meant, which is that those brothers spent the last three years molesting her at every chance. There are other missing parts of the story, too. Like how her father has stopped coming around. And the guy her mother was dating—the one Mom ended up taking care of for nearly two years after he was paralyzed in an accident, bathing him and dressing him and cooking for him before and after work, practically forgetting that Brenda was even there. The guy who, after all that, couldn't take it anymore and so on a hot June morning in the back of Brenda's house put a gun to his head and ended it for good.

If there's one type of kid guaranteed to get her buttons pushed in the wild, it's the one most in need of control. The bugs, the dirt, the wind, and the heat are getting to Brenda in a big way, as if they were conspiring to make her life miserable. At one point she looks at her fingernails, which only a week ago were perfectly painted with lavender nailpolish, notices the first chip, and breaks down in tears. "And how am I supposed to take a bath?" she wails. "I've never been without a shower for more than two days in my life!" The world she so painstakingly built over the past five years, the one she's had under such fierce control, is falling apart in this godforsaken wilderness; elbow to elbow with a bunch of people she cares nothing about, and to her way of thinking has nothing in common with. There is rage and anguish in her eyes, and every now and then, just for a second, a fear like something trapped in a corner and ready to strike.

The first shred of hope comes when she starts whining about it being hot, asks why we can't hike at night instead. Actually, many of the other girls have been asking the same thing, and the staff has already decided to do just that. The rest of the day is spent doing curriculum, working on student growth books, building fires. Brenda takes on the fire-making task with surprising energy. At first I figure her enthusiasm is part of a fantasy that if she blows the right whistles and rings the right bells, maybe they'll let her out of this terrible place early. It turns out to be something more basic. During break, when I notice her not eating, she says one of her biggest horrors of this entire experience is the fact that she's supposed to count whenever she goes to the bathroom. So offensive is the very idea of such a thing, especially when she needs to do serious business, that she's concocted an outrageous plan to eat almost nothing at all, and thus not create any waste until she makes it to buffalo, at which point she'll be free to go to the bathroom without counting. When I seem incredulous, tell her it's hard for me to imagine anyone not going to the bathroom for two or three weeks, she flashes a rankled look; clearly, she plans to make buffalo a whole lot sooner than that.

It's tonight that Brenda does her sitdown in the middle of the road, cursing and spitting at us, driving many of the other girls to new levels of outrage. In the days to come she'll be described by even the most seasoned staff as one of the toughest kids they've seen in a long time. Dave Gahtan says she reminds him of an incredibly stubborn girl some years back who refused to eat or drink for three days. Just before she was about to be hauled out of the program she freaked, started throwing cans of peaches at everybody, then took off in a blind, raging run across the desert. It was one of the few times Dave has had to physically subdue a kid. "She laid on the ground for about ten minutes, and then, for whatever reason, she calmed down and walked back to camp." From then on, she started dealing with her stuff. Dave says she had the most awesome bullshit detector he'd ever seen—could spot kids hiding out, not being honest, from a mile away. Turns out she was one of the best students they'd ever had. Who knows? I think, though I don't really believe it: Maybe Brenda will turn out just like that.

After crawling into bed last night around two o'clock, exhausted from Brenda's angry sitdown, we're awakened just after dawn by a camp full of horse lovers a quarter mile away who've decided to start the day with an hour's worth of cowboy songs blaring from the stereo of their pickup. My eyes pop open to the sound of "That's How the West Was Won," wafting up Rock Creek and across the greasewood flats. Just as I'm thinking there could be nothing more bizarre, Marty Robbins comes on, crooning about that guy with a big iron on his hip, then about the señorita down in the West Texas town of El Paso, in whose arms the storyteller dies after being shot in the chest by the law. Come to think of it, an awful lot of what those guys are singing about—living life alone, running from the law, drinking, and dying—isn't that different from Group 3 after all. The girls may not like the melodies, but add a few horses to our outfit and we're there.

During breakfast the riders come thundering up the wash on four horses and two mules, jackets flying, hands on their hats, whooping like rodeo cowboys. The girls watch, some intrigued but others incredulous. "I don't get it," says Heather. "It's Saturday. Why would anyone spend their weekend out here in the middle of nowhere?"

Food fantasies are back with a vengeance, overtaking our lives. Every one of the girls has a long list of the things she'll eat when she gets out of here, and some run on for several pages. Susan's has grown to 146 items, and includes everything from the usual fast-food fodder to strawberry pancakes at Perkins, frozen yogurt, and her grandma's apple pie. Carla is taking the whole idea one step farther, using food analogies to describe her personality. "Basically, I see myself like a s'more," she tells me. "Brittle, hard graham cracker exterior, the gooey, messy stuff next, and a marshmallow interior, soft and vulnerable." Last week she described to Pam a feeling she was having as being like a "sticky taffy apple." Maybe the therapists could make something of this—develop an entire counseling strategy around food metaphors, explore ways for the kids to build character by mixing ingredients, transform behaviors by steaming and stirring, slicing and dicing. It's worked with nature images for thousands of years—the autumn of life and all that, the seeds of rebirth. Maybe the time has come for a little sugar, some french fries, and a Cuisinart.

I spend a lot of time today talking with Carla. Pam's encouraging her to be more open with the group about her struggles with her family, especially her mother, but in truth she's plain scared to do it. On the other hand, she really wants to be an eagle, and given the leadership responsibilities expected of a kid at that level, making it depends to some extent on how willing she is to be plugged in to the rest of the kids. One of the things you have to do to become an eagle is to call a group on something you feel needs to be dealt with; it remains to be seen whether Carla will choose something of consequence or take the safe route, tossing out an issue closer to salon than therapy. Like I've said, Carla knows she's different from most of the rest of the girls, a member of a world that seems skewed a few degrees off standard orbit. Feeling vulnerable when you're different, she's told me, is more than just paranoia.

Those who've actually talked with Carla's mother say she's a handful. Mistrustful, controlling, fast to blame, uneasy with the world in general. What finally pushes Carla to bite the bullet and share her relationship with her mom is something Pam says, about how many of Carla's own coping styles seem to be the very same ones her mother uses. Evidentially the comment has enough truth in it to scare the hell out of her.

She calls her group in late afternoon, when the heat is down and sun lies thick on the sides of our faces. For a long time she just sits in the circle, eyes to the ground. Finally she starts telling the story of how she ended up here—a tale that, amazingly, even after six weeks, none of the other girls have ever heard.

"I know a lot of you wondered if there wasn't more to how I got here than I've told you. Well, there is. It has to do with my mother. Right now I'm really afraid to go home. I'm afraid to be around her again, her energy. I don't know how I'm supposed to prepare for something like that.

"I didn't come here just because of drugs," she says quietly. "It was a lot because of my anger." Despite weeks of all the girls being prompted by staff to look people in the eyes when talking, Carla's face is to the ground; this time, though, no one says a word. "I've hit my mother. Plenty. I've spit in her face. The last time we were having this huge fight in the car, on the way to school. And I started hitting her. Hard, with my fists. After I got out she called the police—they came and hauled me out of class, charged me with assault. I had a choice of coming here or going to this special home for the next two years."

The rest of the group has some tough questions for her: What's she getting out of the fighting? What's the rest of her family doing to help? What can she do when she gets home to keep from buying into it? In all, though, the other girls are re- markably supportive. Eccentric or not, Carla is part of the tribe; somebody confused and afraid, just like they've been, most of them too many times to count.

It goes on for nearly two hours; by late evening staff has made the decision to move Carla to eagle. The next day, on a glassy morning full of sun, so calm that even the leaves on the cottonwoods have lost their whisper, Jenna comes up behind Carla and blindfolds her, leads her to the site of the transition ceremony, in the shade of an enormous boulder. The girls re- sponsible for designing the ceremony ask me to come along, tell a story, something that might have some special meaning for Carla. I end up settling on an African tale, from the savanna near the Zaire River—Luba country.

A long time ago there was a single, powerful bird liv- ing on a vast, grassy plain, and no one knew her name. Over the years the bird gave birth to lots of children—so many that the day came when there wasn't enough food for them all. So the mother bird called her children around and told them they would have to leave their home to find a better place, a more abundant place. They took hold of her feathers, and with great sweeps of her wings the mother bird rose into the air.

In time the children grew tired of holding on. The hummingbird looked down and saw gardens of beautiful flowers. "That will be home for me," she said, and she let go of her mother's breast and flew down to settle in this new place. Likewise the little kokodyo spotted clusters of fruit trees below, and she too let loose her mother's feathers and dropped down to make a new home on her own. And so it went: the pepper bird coming to rest in a beautiful forest; the desert pelican in patches of wild olives; the secretary bird settling among the termite hills. Until all the young birds had found homes where they could prosper and bear children of their own. The great mother bird climbed very high then, soaring for hours in that blue African sky.

Carla smiles, looks to be breathing it in. On the surface, I tell her, this is a tale about kids severing ties with their parents, about the need at some point to let go of mother to begin a life of their own. But there's another way to look at it, too. Some say each of us is a mother bird, and the young holding onto our feathers are our ideas, our creations. That the time will come when we'll have to carry those ideas, those precious, fragile parts of ourselves, to places where they can prosper and grow— when we'll have to cast them into the lives of the people around us. You have such clever, beautiful ideas, I tell Carla. Your poems, the songs you've been writing and singing to us out here in the desert. These are your gifts to the village. These are your children.

Next the girls tell her what it means to be an eagle. Elizabeth reads a poem she wrote. Finally Jenna takes hold of Carla's arm, opens her hand, places the eagle bead in her palm, and closes her fingers around it. Carla takes off her blindfold and looks around—out into the desert, then at each of us, smiles and wipes tears from her eyes. "This is so cool, you guys," she says. "I'll never forget it. I swear, I'll never forget."

Robert Bly once told an interviewer that an adult is someone who can take the random events and emotions of life and make a story out of them, invest them with meaning. If he's right, at least on this one perfect desert afternoon, Carla seems a little closer to being all grown up.

CHAPTER NINE

LIGHTS OF PASSAGE

IN TRUTH I came here expecting to see ritual, ceremony—slow, beaming moments like Carla's transition to eagle. Moments so full of taste and sensation they can't help but sink into you like a stone; the kind of learning you can ignore but never forget.

Fifteen years ago I was living in southwest Colorado, partway through a hard stumble trying to come to terms with the death of my father, when I fell in with a properly bearded, backcountry-loving therapist who was organizing what for lack of any appropriate term from our own culture can only be called a vision quest. Groups of no more than ten people were getting together, once, maybe twice a year, each of them screened by Doctor Bill to make sure they were every bit as serious as he was. As powerful as nature was for me, I'd never ever been inclined to make my forays into the wilderness acts of community. I signed up less out of faith than desperation.

We spent nearly two months together, one night a week, getting ready, coming to terms with what it was we were trying to do, who we were trying to become; that, in turn, led to eight days of intense, careful ritual in the wild about a hundred miles east of here, outside Canyonlands National Park. I'll skip the details. Suffice it to say it was the one thing that finally allowed me to say good-bye to my father, to slip off the heavy bag of regrets, to celebrate the parts of him that are parts of me.

They told us right from the start that the hardest thing would be coming back. It was. And not just for the obvious reason of going from the exceptional, the beautiful, to the mundane. More troubling by far was that there was simply no context, no language with which to root such passage in the culture at large. For better or worse we were the children of four hundred years of linear thinking, baptized and bottle-fed on notions about the worth of being rational, about the sweetness of being clever, about the prudence of turning our backs on things that we can never fully understand. I was horrified at the thought of being stuck trying to explain the experience to someone and see their eyes glaze over, have them think it was all little more than another feel-good foray into the murky, bullshit-ridden ether of some New Age movement. Mostly I kept my mouth shut.

Still, it haunted me, this notion of ritual, this art of painting footsteps on the dance floor to guide you face-first into the teeth of a change you never asked for. I began exploring the concept of rites of passage, ultimately working with a gifted therapist from California named Kathleen Wall. Doctor Wall had by then

spent years helping clients in her private practice use secular
ritual of their own making as a tool for passing through all kinds
of transitions, a catalyst for getting to the other side of divorce
or the death of a loved one, for knitting stepfamilies together or
for changing careers, for confronting everything from marriage
to birth to the empty nest.

We worked off and on together for nearly two years, ex-
amining the component parts of ritual, looking at the kinds of
rites that had danced entire cultures for centuries. And along
the way we rediscovered some intriguing patterns. The lion's
share of the world's rites of passage, it would appear, were
launched with four basic intentions: the letting go of an old way
of being or an old identity; the acknowledgment or acceptance
of a wandering time—a time when everything's unclear, when
nothing makes sense; the glimpsing of a new self; and finally,
the rooting of a new way of being—a midwifing of new identity
by anchoring it in the culture at large. The really interesting
thing was that when we held up those intentions to certain
developmental theories emerging in psychology, it was a near
perfect fit. We may call them stages. We may tend to think of
them in linear terms though they're clearly not. But to the extent
those therapies work at all, they do so in large part by putting
new clothes on that ancient body of understanding.

One hot afternoon outside Kathleen's house in San Jose
we were talking about how ritual figures in the lives of young
people. Adolescents especially, she said, are hungry for rites of
passage. That was pretty much the opposite of what I'd always
assumed, having long noticed their boredom, even disdain for
things like bar mitzvahs and high school graduations. "If you
don't give young people meaningful rituals," she said, "—and
meaning is the key—they'll create them on their own. Look at

gangs. The colors and the special clothes, the language, the in-
itiation challenges, the rules of behavior. That's ritual in the
most basic sense: communal action, intended to empower by
anchoring a sense of new identity.''

It's only since I've come to this program that I'm finally
seeing some of that kid hunger Kathleen Wall was talking about.
Graduating from coyote to buffalo or buffalo to eagle might to
some seem cute at best, to others, hopelessly simpleminded. But
standing here in this wild country, stripped of convention,
where over time it begins to be okay to feel and say things
without having to worry about being cool, where the land is
the primary witness and the land does not make judgments of
you, plays no favorites, where in this smudged, greasy-haired
tribe there is a hint of community and in that small glimpse a
sudden hunger for more of it—then is when the real power of
ritual comes home to roost.

On the bad days I wonder if it's worth gaining vision in
the first place if the folks back home can't provide you with a
place for it, if you're left stumbling around with yearning in your
back pocket and no clue what to do with it. Too often in this
culture coming home from an honest-to-goodness rite of passage, having touched something that truly inspired, can be a
terrible thing. Maybe the only thing worse is having never
touched it at all.

CHAPTER TEN

MAKING FOR THE MOUNTAIN

THE GIRLS ABOUT to graduate from Group 3 are bouncing off
the walls. I've seen squirrels with less twitch. Sara and Lisa are
pissed at the thought of having to go to a therapeutic boarding
school. Jenna, on the other hand—strong, Xena warrior of the
desert—is increasingly scared about going home, back to the
same old friends, the same temptations. "I just hope I can say
no," she tells us over and over. On top of that Nancy is put out
with Lisa for ditching her friends to try to flirt with one of the
instructors, and the two of them end up out at the edge of camp
locked in a yell fest for almost an hour.

The good news is a slight shift in Brenda, who seems actually to be using her acid tongue to build relationships with

some of the staff instead of simply skewering them with it. She's especially happy to engage Steve, though it takes him a while to recognize her commentaries as peace offerings. I watch him this afternoon, encouraged when Brenda smiles and agrees with him that yes, you can find good clothes at the Gap, undone soon after, when he tells her he bought the shirt he has on at a sale at JC Penney.

"No wonder you look so tacky," she tells him, then proceeds to ask if he ever takes showers. Over the next fifteen minutes the two of them talk about the food we're eating—"What am I supposed to do for a decent meal around here—go out and kill a deer or something?"—then circle around to her being on suicide watch, which she knows full well is a consequence of always talking about dying, part of her ongoing effort to push buttons. She's definitely getting tired of sleeping under a tarp with two people on either side of her, let alone having female staff within arm's reach with their backs turned every time she has to go to the bathroom. Of course she wouldn't be much of a chess player if she let her frustration show. "You know," she tells Steve at the end of the break. "If I wasn't so lazy I'd get up three or four times at night to go to the bathroom just to piss you guys off."

One other piece of hopeful news. As we do every day right before hitting the trail, this morning we circled up with backpacks on and did a feelings check—a simple matter of going around the group and everyone tossing out a one-liner about what kind of mood they're in: I feel anxious, I feel sad, whatever. When it got to Susan she paused, told us she was about to say something she'd never said before. "I feel happy," she announced with a grin. We all applauded.

There was a time not so long ago, when spring got sufficiently full of itself to melt the snows in the high country, that the kids would begin a marvelous trek west, away from the Henrys, passing through the eight-mile-wide band of water-pocket folds that form the spine of Capitol Reef National Park, up into the Douglas fir, the ivory-colored stands of aspen on Boulder Mountain. Dry to wet, low to high, looking down, where in the weeks before it was mostly looking up. Those who've done it talk of it like it was a march to the Elysian fields.

No more. Now we load the kids into Suburbans, put blindfolds on them to cut them off from any view of the traffic, the motels, the Subway sandwich shop and the Exxon in Torrey, roar them through the park, and drop them off at a trailhead on the east side of Boulder Mountain. All this in large part because some kids in another program, here under court orders, got loose in the park, stole a few things, including a truck. Lots of complaints, the Park Service says. "You know it's one thing to have these kids roaming around in the backcountry," a guy in Torrey tells me. "But we can't have them harassing the public." An eight-mile walk in a remote part of the park, four staff for eight kids, not a single overnight. All I can say is thank God for all this plug-ugly Bureau of Land Management land where no one seems to want to go—that, and a mountain full of timber which isn't all that popular either, at least not yet—where we can hide our thugs and hooligans should, God forbid, someone come down the trail.

It's a tiresome, irritating ride to the trailhead at Grouse Creek; understandably the girls are doing everything they can to peek out from behind the blindfolds. "But it's so pretty," Nancy protests, right before Tricia lets out a delighted scream on spying the Subway. Karen—the escort I went to Salt Lake City with to pick up Kevin, Keith, and Susan—is driving, and she's obviously thrilled to see the kids again, smiling over them in the rearview mirror as if she were their favorite aunt picking them up after a month at summer camp.

Fifteen minutes after climbing out of the rig at Grouse Creek, sweet now with the vanilla smell of ponderosa and the pepper scent of aspen coming back to life, we're on the trail again, heading for camp. Brenda, in one of the first displays of emotion I've ever seen in her, tells me that she likes it here on the mountain—is smiling over it, saying how the smell of pine reminds her of home. Nancy must like coming to the mountain, too, because tonight after dinner, five weeks from the day she first came into the field, she finally finds the courage to tell the full story of her dance with bulimia to the group. "I feel weak talking about it," she says, "and I don't like feeling weak. The thing is, though, I trust all you guys." Who knows, maybe being here in the forest is somehow soothing to her—a maze of hiding places just beyond the firelight, a world of darkness within easy reach.

Her story begins with memories of the third grade, being "a little chunk." By the time Nancy reached eleven her mother was concerned enough with her weight—and in particular, how the other kids would treat her because of it—that she drove Nancy out to a strip mall and enrolled her in a diet program. She says it probably didn't help that she grew up in Florida, on a beach, where there were always lots of beautiful people running around in bathing suits.

"The next year—I was in seventh grade—a friend told me

about throwing up, so I started that. I did it all the time. Always. My life has been one big lie.''

Nancy goes on to tell us that her parents pretty much turned their backs on the throwing up; they didn't see it because they didn't want to. "We're supposed to be these perfect children, and anything we do to lessen that image isn't talked about or dealt with.''

Over time she got so she didn't care what her parents thought about anything. She got high, stole a car, drove north to Atlanta, where she wrecked it. "They came and got me," she tells us, tears beginning to show in the firelight. "They took me home. Not a word was said. Not to this day.''

Jenna wants to know what it feels like to be bulimic. "It's a high," Nancy says. "It's a wonderful high, and I love it. Yogurt and ice cream are the best. Besides, if I didn't have it I'm pretty sure my life would fall apart." She pauses for a couple of seconds. "I have to say something to you guys. When I first meet someone, it doesn't matter who or where, my first thought is that they must figure I'm the ugliest, fattest person in the world. This is the first place I've ever been where people seem to really care about me. That's never happened before, and before I got here, I didn't trust it. I wasn't used to that. I feel more at home here than at home.''

In all it's the kind of self-portrait that will leave Pam with her work cut out for her, trying to prod Mom and Dad to take a look at some good eating-disorder clinics Nancy can go to when she gets out of here. Bulimia is a thorny problem, and she's clearly far enough into it to need some expert help. Besides, after years spent hinting about the problem but getting little reaction, at least at a clinic she'll be surrounded by people who know enough to take her seriously.

The next morning Brenda overhears us talking about the fact
that anyone who manages to build a fire with a pine spindle on
a pine board gets a pound of M&M's. She's going to make it
happen, by God, and that means today. Never mind that she's
only built three fires with a sage set, and the difference between
that and pine-on-pine is sort of like landing a Cessna on a mile
of runway compared to setting a jet down on an aircraft carrier;
the same principles are at work, but one takes a whole lot more
finesse. Like a lot of kids, Brenda has almost no patience for
long journeys around the learning curve. If something takes
more than five minutes of sheer will or muscle, then who the
hell needs it anyway. Some might call that ADD. But in Brenda's
case it seems more a matter of seeing early failures as a sign of
being a screw-up. Stay with what you're naturally good at, don't
go beyond the edge of your current abilities, and life will give
you a lot less pain.

Fortunately, just minutes after she makes the decision to
go pine-on-pine, Lavoy shows up—out of nowhere, of course—
like some kind of guardian angel, ends up helping her put a set
together. All the while he's talking, teaching, asking her why
rotten wood might not work as well as good wood, what difference it would make to change the shape of the spindle point.
She gives it a quick, furious try and gets nothing, flies into a
rage, and then sits down in the dirt in a huff. "You know, the
people who take the longest time getting this thing to work are
the ones who end up knowing the most about it," Lavoy tells
her. "Things being easy isn't always the best recipe for success,
or knowledge, or even happiness." He goes on to talk about a
family of kids he taught in school who weren't academically

gifted at all, always struggling. They got into wrestling, he says, they grew to love it, and that made all the difference. Suddenly they were willing to put in the effort to get decent grades because they knew they had to to keep doing the thing they loved.

If Brenda is still fighting, Susan continues on most days to stay out of the hole. "This place is so much better than a hospital," she tells me, though she doesn't give the same reasons other kids do—that in a hospital you can manipulate the system, figure out what the therapists want to see, give them exactly that, then go back to distracting yourself with television and computer games. Susan's description of the suicide ward is a lot like her description of school. "There are so many people there," she explains. "That makes it way too easy to hide. It's the troublemakers that end up getting all the attention, and the rest of the kids just end up laying low, trying not to stick out. Out here in the woods I get to figure out stuff on my own. I've got a lot more power over what kind of day I'm gonna have."

Late in the morning I notice Lisa at the edge of camp, sitting by herself, and that almost never happens. Besides browbeating Josh a couple of weeks back for acting more like a parent to the group than a buddy, as if he were on some sort of power trip, of late Lisa's most cherished rant has been against the whole idea of therapy; given that she's leaving tomorrow, heading off to graduation, I ask if she'd be willing to sit and talk about what the big terrible deal is. She agrees, and we take a seat in a blanket of pine needles under a big ponderosa. At first she doesn't say anything—just stares off into the woods, as if settling her emotions enough to stitch together some kind of thoughtful critique instead of just handing me another bucket of outrage. For that alone I'm proud of her. A few weeks back, outrage is all she would have been able to offer. Evidently a couple of hundred "I

feel" statements over the past eight weeks—the structured format the kids use to express their emotions in group—has had
some effect after all.

"Okay," she says. "The whole therapy thing—it can be
good. Some of it can help. But too often it's like a religion. Like
a cult. People get so devoted to the theory of it, and that's the
only filter they ever use. They can only connect to you through
the theory. It's like if you have something terrible happen to
you, and you tell some superreligious person, and all she can
say is, 'Well, God knows best.' That's not understanding somebody. It's not even trying. It's just putting the world into boxes."

It's probably worth noting that Lisa has a penchant for
picking fights, for maneuvering in ways that let her maintain her
sense of power, getting the last word or the final sour look; it's
a safe bet that even the best therapists would have their hands
full trying to stay ahead of her. I imagine it must be next to
impossible to keep her from stuffing you into her own box of
preconceived notions she's built about anyone in an authority
position. Plain and simple, if you have any say over what happens in Lisa's life, the odds are against you.

"So what are you going to do when you get back to boarding school?" I ask her. "A week from now you'll be in that
whole scene again."

"Look," she says, "I've learned this much since I've been
down here. It was a mistake to fight battles I couldn't win. Small
stuff, mostly. Just not saying anything isn't necessarily the same
thing as compromising my values, my personal truth. If I say
something opposite of what I think, that I can't live with. But
there's something to be said for playing the game when I have
to—even then, though, only to a point."

Like many of the girls, Lisa wants to know what the boys

of Group 4 have been up to, so I tell her about the poetry slams, about how everybody gets respect when they read their stuff around the fire. She's impressed, says that kind of support is hard to come by.

"There's something you should know," she tells me. "I learned more in the first week and a half out here than in a year and a half of therapy. For one thing, people are more real here. They've got this whole big variety of ideas and experiences to share—they're not all coming from the same religion, the same set of theories. They're thinking for themselves. Besides, look around you. It takes work to live out here like this. You can't wait around for someone else to take care of you."

We sit in silence for a few minutes. Across camp Brenda is trying to bust out a pine-on-pine fire again. Jenna is working on a ghost bead necklace for her sister. Susan sits against a tree, head hung over her lap, scribbling in her journal.

"Seems like you've been awfully upset with your parents," I say to Lisa. "I'm wondering—looking back, what is it you think they did wrong? Where'd they drop the ball?"

She flashes a hard look, takes a breath, lets it go. "I just don't think you should ignore a kid who's so sad, who's been miserable for such a long time. Just send her away."

"But I thought you asked to be sent away," I say.

"Yeah, well, that was a year and a half ago. I've got siblings, you know. I'd kind of like to grow up with them." She looks away, lets out a long sigh. "I don't know," she adds, sounding weary. "I'm sure they're trying their best."

A light rain begins to fall. I'm just about to thank her, get up and go over to check on Brenda, when she gives me the strangest look. For a split second those proud, defiant eyes of hers turn into something else altogether—the eyes of somebody

a lot sadder, a lot more worn out than you'd think was possible
at fifteen.

"It's just that I'm so tired of the staff at school coming up
to me and saying, 'Lisa, what I think you might want to work
on,' or 'This is what I see going on with you,' whenever I do
something silly. I mean it's work on this, work on that. C'mon,
I was fourteen years old! Sometimes you just need to live.
There's this notion of perfection—that's my parents' ideal. But
I don't believe in perfection. They're interested in results. Well,
I'm not a result. I'm a friggin' human being."

The radio call from backup comes, saying the truck will
be here to pick up graduates in about two hours—much earlier
than we expected. We hustle to stitch a couple of tarps together
for a good-bye group, manage to circle up just as the north wind
kicks in and the clouds break loose for real. There we are, hanging off the side of Boulder Mountain in a huddle of ponderosa
pine, staff and students crushed together into this gaggle of wool
and Gore-Tex, wet hands and faces, some of it from the weather,
some from tears.

Both the field staff and the therapists start working with kids
weeks before they leave, prompting them to play out in their
heads the kinds of situations likely to come up on home turf,
encouraging them to shore up their plans for how to cope. At
the same time the therapists are talking with parents about plans
for aftercare, which can include everything from Alcoholics
Anonymous or Narcotics Anonymous meetings, therapy, finding
a job, changing schools, even moving to another town. But for
all that, in truth there's probably no such thing as adequately

preparing a kid to make the shift from this safe, nomadic existence in the arms of the wilderness to life back home.

Several of the girls tell Jenna they're worried about her— not if she can make things happen, but whether she can keep believing she can. Three months ago she was a gang-banger wannabe, locked in a relationship with a guy who beat her, gasping for air in a sea of cocaine and booze and heroine. And then in that desert, and on this mountain, so strong and vibrant, an incredible athlete who on more than one occasion plucked the pack off a sick girl and tossed it onto her own, trekked up the road with seventy-five pounds on her back like there were rockets on her feet. Still, this emerging leader taking charge of life is a new role for her. To the rest of us it's perfect casting, but there are days when she doesn't trust it. Jenna's family can't afford aftercare. On Friday, for better or worse, she's heading home.

"You're so loyal," one of the instructors tells her. "Such a good, loyal friend. I'm scared for you that this loyalty is going to work against you, that you'll choose loyalty to your friends over loyalty to yourself."

"I worry about that too," Jenna says.

All the time this is going on, Brenda sits back with a look of disdain on her face. Staff prompts her to offer something to the group, but all she can say is that she doesn't know any of these people, and so their going away really doesn't mean much to her. Afterward she'll ask me what's wrong with the staff, all of them so stressed about these kids leaving. "Why would you get attached to people you know are going to leave?" she asks, genuinely confounded. "It's stupid to involve yourself with something you know will cause you pain."

"What about your father?" I ask. "You told me he's cut you out of his life, but that you still like seeing him—it bothers you that he hasn't called for such a long time."

"He can do whatever he likes," she says, bristling. "It doesn't matter to me one way or another."

CHAPTER ELEVEN

IN THE COUNCIL OF BABA FATS

WHEN I WAS little, maybe seven or eight, I used to have the strangest recurring dream. There was no plot, no story—just walking slowly through a half-darkened living room, stopping to gaze at something—a chair, a couch—and getting so focused on it that it seemed as if I could feel the pulse of the thing, this odd, clocklike throbbing that would finally grow so intense I'd wake up in a puddle of sweat. I hadn't thought of it for years. Out with the boys of Group 4 again, sometimes there's a similar, almost unbelievable intensity oozing through our days—life under a magnifying glass, enlarging every move we make, every conversation, turning up the volume of our minutes, be they anxious or sublime, until we become hyperaware of everything.

It's ritual at sixty miles an hour, and the only time it stops is early in the morning when you're the only one awake, lying in your bag with your wool hat on, right before dawn gives shape back to the world.

Sort of like today, when Kevin comes over to tell us that somebody ripped off his peaches and a bag of ramen. In the real world such a theft might leave you a little hot under the collar. Out here it's everything. We grind to a halt and circle up and talk and wait for someone to come clean, and when no one does we sit in silence a good forty-five minutes; if the sun weren't growing hotter on the backs of our necks and the patches of shade shifting on the ground around us, there'd be no indication the world was turning at all. All of us stuck for eternity in this moment, waiting for the confession of a teenage thief. Finally Shawn, the senior instructor, speaks up—clearly he's pissed. And since Shawn doesn't turn up the heat very often, when he does even the slackers pay attention.

"I'm so tired of this shit," he says, his voice fairly compelling the kids to listen. "You guys have done well for the most part with the carts, with opening up emotionally—with poetry and groups. But the stealing, the cussing, the derogatory references to women—I'm tired of it. We try to give you options, and we end up getting screwed. That's fine. If you can't handle leniency, then we'll try something different.

"You guys don't get it. You lie here, you'll lie back home. You steal here, and you'll steal back home. You can't communicate with each other here, you can't communicate back home. This isn't just about peaches and ramen. You go home and screw up on a job or in school, you want one more try, well, sooner or later someone is going to say to hell with you."

As would be a common consequence for any staff to dish

out, Shawn tells the group that the theft means no peaches or ramen for anyone next week, which in the outside world is about like saying no television or car keys. Then he calls the staff away from the group, leaving the boys to try to persuade the guilty party to come clean, which he never does.

We walk long and hard today—whether by the simple need to make miles or from an effort to hike the bullshit out of the boys, it's hard to say. Come nightfall we're well into the outer edges of the Red Desert, and some two hours later, in the heart of it, entering through a narrow-slot canyon of chocolate-colored rock, a shocking, moonlit portal leading into the bleakest, loneliest basin I've ever seen. Not a tree anywhere, and on the ground, scattered patches of alkali stains from a ribbon of foul water meandering across the bottoms. No sound other than a warm, fitful wind screaming down the walls. No one has the energy to cook, so we go hand-to-mouth with granola, break off a few hunks of cheese, pour down some truly god-awful water, crawl into our bags, and call it a night.

Again, vivid dreams. This time I'm standing on the porch of a large home beside a lake, milling around with a bunch of what seem to be wealthy, somewhat snobbish people. At one point I look up to see a middle-aged man walking along the shore of the lake. He stops, takes off his shoes, and swims out to the middle, where he takes off the rest of his clothes, then sinks down through the clear water to the bottom, apparently trying to kill himself. No one else seems moved to do anything, so I rush down to the shore, struggle to remove layer after layer of my own clothes, finally manage to dive in and set about trying to rescue him. Once at the bottom, the guy has turned into a teenage girl. I drag her out to the shore, where she coughs and sputters but recovers. The last I see of her she's in the big house,

off the living room, making a call to a guy she used to go with
who beat her, trying her best to get back together with him.
There's this sour lump in the pit of my stomach.

Monday morning, end of the road for Larry, Wade, Frank, and
Ray, who'll be taken out of the field later today to a site at the
edge of the desert. There, along with graduates from the other
groups, they'll spend the next two days talking about going
home, about how they're going to deal with old issues, finally
link up with their families toward the end of the week. We have
a good-bye group for them at the base of an enormous sandstone
wall some two hundred feet high, pock-marked with erosion
holes the size of watermelons. The whole time a pair of ravens
wing high above us, peeling back and forth across the upper
reaches of the cliff.

   We go around the circle and everyone shares something
with the guys who are leaving—memories, best wishes, fears
for their future. Then the grads do the same thing back. Wade
recites his favorite poem, which has been an underground classic around here for years—a sharp little ramble by Shel Silver-
stein called "The Perfect High." The story centers on a kid
named Gimmesome Roy, whose sole purpose in life is to try
every drug imaginable, searching for the ultimate buzz. One day
he hears about a guru living on a mountaintop in Nepal, a guy
named Baba Fats, who supposedly knows the secret to the perfect high. Inspired, Gimmesome Roy spends the next fourteen
years searching for the guru, knocking himself senseless climbing the mountain, finally makes it, "coughing blood . . . aching
and shaking and weak." When Baba Fats tells him that the perfect high lies within himself, Gimmesome Roy goes ballistic,

calls him a jive motherfucker, rails on about how he didn't
spend fourteen years getting up that mountain to listen to crap;
says if Baba doesn't tell him the real secret he'll kill him. So Fats
invents this outrageous tale about how the perfect high comes
from the tzu-tzu flower, which grows in a distant land beyond
the River Slime, a wretched place guarded by a nasty witch and
mucous beasts and a one-eyed giant. Gimmesome Roy breaks
into tears of joy, then walks off down the mountain to find it.

"Well, that is that," says Baba Fats, sitting back down on his stone,
   facing another thousand years of talking to God alone.
"It seems, O Lord," says Baba Fats, "they're all the same: old men
   or bright-eyed youth.
"It's always easier to sell them some shit than it is to give them
   the truth."

When the group finally winds down, Frank, our brilliant,
beat-style poet, is to everyone's amazement on the verge of
tears. Shawn and Jesse are holding their breath, wanting him to
let go, let it out just once, but he maintains, in the end decides
to speak to us as a group. "I've always thought good-bye was
an oxymoron," he says. "You're my friends. What else can I say?
You're my friends. That's perfect."

It would have been a total love fest had Brad not shown
up, telling the boys that unless the person who stole the peaches
and ramen confesses, the truck coming to pick up the grads will
be sent back. "Wade, Larry, Ray, and Frank—you guys will have
to forgo participating in any of the grad activities. We'll take you
out of the field at the end of the week, at the last minute." Also,
for the rest of the group, only staple foods next week. No brown
sugar, no peaches, ramen, granola. No hot chocolate or cider.

"We'll leave you guys alone to work it out. It's up to you." And with that the staff gets up and moves fifty yards down the road.

If Brad's intent was to provoke a riot, he's done a masterful job. Larry breaks into uncontrolled sobs, and Wade is cussing a blue streak. At one point Wade sees some of the staff looking at the group and he shouts at us. "Quit fucking looking at us! That's not in the rules!" At which point Brad calmly walks over, talks to them about their language for what must be the tenth time this week, and walks away. Fifteen minutes later fourteen-year-old Ruben comes over to us, says he's the one who stole the food.

We're shocked. Most of us thought the thief was Wade. In fact Shawn and Jesse confronted him about it in private yesterday, at which point he flatly denied it and walked off in a huff. Everyone is congratulating Ruben on having the guts to say something, while Kate and I are trying to swallow the lump in our throats we feel at having quietly been pointing the finger at the wrong kid. "It means more to me that you apologized than that you stole the peaches," Kevin says. Later Brad pulls Ruben aside, questions him about the details of the theft, seems satisfied by his account. Next week, though, we'll learn that it was Wade all along, that Ruben figured he'd earn some brownie points with the guys by taking the fall; Brad will be so outraged he'll call Wade up at home and try to talk him into giving his eagle bead back.

For now, though, Ruben's confession is enough. The truck sent to pick up the grads has been waiting a half mile down the road. It gets the radio call. We pile in; the driver makes a U-turn and sends us flying across the desert in a cloud of dust.

A former instructor named Jim, a calm man about forty, is running the grad site, and his first challenge is to convince Wade, Frank, and Ray that they need to go to the creek and clean up a bit. "It's not a bad thing that you're dirty," Jim says. "But hey, we have to think of the impact you guys will have on the parents. We don't want to scare them." While the guys are rummaging around in their packs, Jim pulls Wade aside, looks at his shredded pants with the boxer shorts showing through, tells him that he needs to change into something else, which for Wade means into the only clothing he has left, shorts. "Can't do, man," Wade says matter-of-factly. "I look like a geek." In the end he talks to Frank, who agrees to help him sew his pants up with some stray pieces of sinew he has in his pack. "Not while they're on you though, man," Frank says. "I don't want to be needling around next to the jewels."

Pretty soon another truck full of graduates pulls in, all of them so centered, polite, and articulate that for a minute I wonder if they're from another program altogether. My boys are ragtags by comparison—hip-hop, outrageous, a bit crude, and the weird thing is that part of me loves them for it; I feel like a parent, comparing my kids with somebody else's, and of course no matter how you cut it, coming up grateful that I landed with the boys of Group 4.

Wednesday morning I've got a little time to myself, decide to kick things off with a big breakfast at Sam's Country Cafe in Loa—relax for a couple of hours, turn it off. I sit at the counter next to the coffeepot, and just as I'm about to take a sip from my first cup I happen to look above the sink and see a poster that seems awfully close to black humor. "Arguing with kids is like wrestling with a pig in the mud," it says. "After a while you realize the pig enjoys it."

The parents and brothers and sisters, even an uncle or two have by now arrived in Loa; most are staying in rooms near base, at the Trout Creek Inn, taking an occasional drive or roaming the streets, riding a roller coaster of excitement and knee-shaking fear about what it will be like to see the enraged, depressed, or defiant kid they last saw two months before. Tonight is the parent meeting, where a therapist will brief the families on what they can expect from Thursday's reunion; when we meet at seven o'clock the anxiety is thick enough to cut with a knife. The only person even close to content is Kristine's seven-year-old brother, Kyle, who's happy as a clam at the thought of seeing his sister, whether she's changed or not.

"You're talking about having these conversations with our kids," Wade's parents tell Paul, the therapist, after the meeting gets started. "But it's been a long time since we've been able to converse with Wade at all." Around the room a dozen heads are bobbing up and down in agreement. To their credit, most of the families profess a willingness to make a fresh start, but not all. "Don't tell me how my kid's gonna act," says one father, angry with all this therapy nonsense. "I think after all these years I know him better than you." Turns out he's one of the parents who promised to go to counseling over the past two months and then blew it off.

The next morning the families meet Lavoy, who turns the conference room of the Trout Creek Inn into a classroom, engaging them in one of the curriculum lessons, delighting them with the chemistry of fire. He starts with a bow-drill, moves deftly into a discussion of photosynthesis, from there on to the combustion of a jet engine, and finally, to the very cells firing within us all. "That Lavoy," I hear one woman saying later. "Oh, if only my teachers would have been like him." Afterward Jim shows up, the guy in charge of the grad site, announces the plan for the rest of the day. He asks that in order to fit better into the world their kids have been living in, would they please forgo jewelry and makeup, as well as any candy, cookies, or other treats they may have brought with them. He further explains that staff will keep all medications, doling them out to parents just as they do for the kids—in part to give Mom and Dad a sense of what the kids went through but, more important, as a matter of safety, just in case somebody with itchy fingers would make off with them. On hearing this, the same father who was bent out of shape last night is even more irritated. "This program was for my kid," he growls, scoffing at the notion that holding his blood-pressure medicine would give him a better sense of what the program felt like. "This is his deal, not mine."

Thirty miles down the highway our nine-car parade comes to a halt when our lead vehicle—one of the infamous Dodge trucks—stalls out in front of the Capitol Reef Visitors Center. The good news is that everyone is so used to breakdowns that they handle the situation like a pit crew at Daytona; Lavoy wheels his pickup around, we push the old Dodge into the parking lot, call base for help, load the essentials into the other truck, and in ten minutes are back on the road again.

The cars are left in a gravel lot along the highway, and we walk a hundred yards up a dirt road to a cluster of pines, roughly a mile and a half downstream from the grad site where the kids have gathered. The therapists are there to circle up the families; they encourage everyone to take a few deep breaths, look around, try to get in touch with the beauty of the place. A surprising number go for it, as if they're eager to take in everything they can about this reunion—turning their faces to the spring sun and the towers of slickrock, praying, I imagine, for a fresh start. Finally Paul walks a few yards off from the group, makes a radio call, comes back with a big grin on his big face. "Here's what we're going to do," he says, sounding very excited himself. "I'm going to hold down the button on this radio, and when I give the signal all of you are going to shout out, 'Are you ready?' When we hear back from the kids, I'll press the button again and we'll all yell, 'On your mark, set, go!' And at that point they'll start moving this direction—some running, a few probably not." He reminds the families to stand together, even divorced parents, so as not to make kids have to choose one family member over another, tells them to be sure to hand off their cameras to a staff person so they can get photos for them; I end up with three in my hands, all from parents of kids I've never met.

More often than not a graduation run-in is a kind of emotional end of the rainbow, a stirring reconnection that leaves even complete strangers with tears streaming down their faces. It's every sappy movie and heart-plinking novel you ever got choked up about, and with a lot of kids, just for a minute you can believe that here is the force of love and longing in helpings big enough to heal the past.

Larry, the kid who couldn't take care of himself, who tried to end it all one way or another by lying down in swirls of sleet and snow in his underwear, is among the first over the line, running down that dirt road with stumbling legs, gasping for breath, collapsing in the arms of his father and mother, tears falling from his parents' faces onto the dusty lenses of his glasses. Kristine is next, true to form the first girl to arrive, kneeling down first to hug her little brother, Kyle, who wraps his arms around her and won't let go so that she ends up having to hug her parents by rising with him still clinging to her for dear life. The hug she gives her father is light, reserved, and when he turns I can see the disappointment in his face. Next comes a fifteen-year-old named Scott, beaming, a kid who woke up this morning and refused his regular dose of the powerful antidepressant Welbutrin—told the staff it made him feel high, disconnected, that this was a special day, a ceremony, and he wanted to be fully present for it.

On it goes, twelve kids in all. Not surprisingly, Wade, Frank, and Ray decide to walk instead of run, ambling three abreast down the road like a trio of gunslingers stripped of their weapons, kids who as a simple matter of cool can't be seen running into their mothers' arms, whether they feel the urge to or not. It goes the worst for Sara, our quirky queen of smudge. She stops six feet from her parents, breaks down in tears, turns her back on them and walks off, crumples into a heap under a giant ponderosa. "Maybe we shouldn't have come," I hear her father say to Lavoy. "Do you think we should go home?"

"She just needs a little time," Lavoy tells her father in a reassuring voice, his hand on his shoulder. "You've probably been in situations where you decided something was right, and the next day you knew that wasn't the move you should have made."

"Yeah," her father says, looking incredibly sad.

"Well, then," Lavoy says. "You just relax, stay right here. There's nothing in this world that can stand up to the force of love. You give her all the love you possibly can—tomorrow's another day, and things will turn around."

By the time it's over my mouth is sore from grinning, my eye hurts from squinting through other people's cameras, and my arms are tired from all the hugging. Somewhat disturbing is an episode involving that irritable father, who after a quick embrace of his graduating son decides to run off and climb a steep dome of slickrock beside the road. Coming down he slips and falls, skins his legs and elbows, leaves his son shaking his head and me wishing that we could haul Dad back to base for processing, trade his Eddie Bauer shorts for a pair of army pants, send him into the desert for a rite of passage of his own.

An hour for lunch—cheese, granola bars, and fruit. Tricia, the chatty, overindulged girl who arrived at base with a trunk full of Clinique, is astonishing her family by eating three apples in a row, core and all. "I don't even sleep on a ground pad anymore," she tells her mother, who looks to be in a mild state of shock. It reminds me of the therapist who got a call from a distraught mother a month after graduation, asking what she should do about her son. "He's sleeping out in the yard. He won't even use his own bed!"

At the end of lunch we start a mile-and-a-half trek back up the same dirt road the kids ran down, heading for the grad site. The families have done their best to comply with the request to bag the jewelry and the makeup; still, most look incredibly out of place. On reaching five-foot-wide Grouse Creek, which consists of barely eight inches of water scattered with stones, some are nearly dumbstruck on how to get across. A few end up flagging down the pickup full of camping gear and begging rides on the tailgate, hopping off on the other side giddy with the thrill of it. It's then I realize that these parents will never be able to comprehend what it is their kids have gone through for the past eight weeks: the sweat and the fear and the stinking water, the cups full of beans shoveled out of blackened billy pots, the climbing of mountains and the stumbling through deserts—life in the raw, with all the horror and thrill that affords.

Dave Gahtan tells of a sixteen-year-old boy graduating last winter, when the place was so full of snow that staff had to shovel out spots on the ground for the families to sleep. At one

point this kid's parents were huddled in a canvas tent, going on
about how horrible this was, saying they couldn't believe their
child had gone through such a thing. Maybe they meant it as a
compliment. Anyway, the boy broke down—just started sobbing. When his alarmed parents asked what was wrong he told
them how much it hurt for them to find this so terrible, when
to him it was the first place in the world where he ever felt
truly connected. He said it was sad to realize how different he
was from them—that to him the most frightening, dangerous
place in the world wasn't here but home.

It's one of the great strokes of genius of this program that
for one night families are given a box of basic foodstuffs, sleeping bags, and tarps, then hiked off by their kids to a solo site in
the woods where their only chance of eating hot food and sleeping warm depends on the skill of those prodigal sons and daughters. How strange for parents, especially the more powerful
fathers and mothers of political and corporate America, to suddenly be forced into giving the reins to kids who eight weeks
ago they wouldn't have trusted with twenty bucks for a bag of
groceries.

Before all that, though, are several hours of initiatives, trust-
building activities, and most significantly, "I feel circles," where
you can call anyone you want into the center of the group to let
them know what's on your mind—take care of old business, tell
your truth. The formula used is one the kids have practiced daily
for two months, and in which the parents got a crash course late
last night: "I feel this way . . . When you do or say . . . I imagine
it's because . . . In the future I'd like to see . . ." Each piece of
what the speaker says is repeated by the listener. The whole purpose of such structure is to keep conversations on track, to help
people rise above their nearly overwhelming urges to snipe at

one another, to fall back onto that he-said-she-said Ferris wheel they've been spinning on for months, even years.

At first our circle is little more than a feel-good festival, tearful parents calling kids in and saying how proud they are, sharing their commitment to making things work at home. Little Kyle, though, Kristine's brother, gets way into it, first calling his sister into the circle to say he loves her, that he imagines that's because he missed her so much, and that in the future he wants to see a lot more of her. He follows this up by calling Josh, the instructor, in, telling him he feels sorry that his truck broke down today on the way to the grad site, that he imagines it's because it's such a nice truck, that in the future he hopes he can get it fixed.

Brad is running the circle, and after an hour of nothing but happy weeping it's clear he's ready to see the group dive under the surface and drag up whatever creepy things may be lying there. Finally he calls Kyle out, tells him that he feels happy that Kyle is participating, but that he's sad that the older people don't have the same courage. Frank is the first to take the hint, blows out a breath, calls his father into the center of the circle.

"I feel sad," Frank says in a quiet voice, "because I don't really know you." He pauses for a minute, and I'm sitting here wondering if he's going to tell his dad what he's told us, that the guy has never given a crap about him—never even sees him other than to pick him up at the airport when he gets kicked out of one boarding school, climb into the car with him again a couple of weeks later after pulling strings to finagle him a spot someplace else. But with his dad sitting here on the ground within arm's reach, looking awkward, breathing hard, red-faced and weak from all the years of drinking, he just can't seem to muster the courage. "I imagine I don't know you because of the big age difference between us," Frank says lamely, looking at Brad, hoping he'll let it pass.

No such luck. "Frank," Brad says, "there are a lot of people here older than you. What is it that makes you want to know this particular man?"

Frank fumbles for another minute, saying how he and his dad have never spent any time together, at which point his father, trashing the ground rules, jumps in and tries to explain. Brad makes a halfhearted attempt to bring him back to the format—reminding him of the need to repeat what Frank just said, but he's too anxious, too much in a hurry to say what he needs to say. At first I wonder if maybe he's just blowing Brad off as a matter of course, the habit of a very powerful man, used to being in charge, who doesn't take kindly to being interrupted by some backwoods therapist in sweat pants and sneakers. But there's an urgency in his voice, a desperation, as if he's standing on the edge of something he's wanted to tell his son for a long time, and that if he doesn't put it out there right this minute God only knows if he'll ever find the courage to do it again. There are tears in his eyes, and both Frank and his mother look utterly shocked.

"Frank, I've made so many mistakes. Your whole life I've been trying to make you into what I wanted you to be, instead of letting you be yourself. That was wrong. It was wrong. I don't know if you can ever forgive me. But I want you to know that I'm sorry. I want you to know that I love you, Frank. I love you." And with that Frank wipes away the first tears to fall down his cheeks in a long, long while, nods at his father, crawls back into his place in the circle, and hangs his head and cries.

Several staff are here who've worked with Frank for the past two months. They've loved this kid, cared deeply about him, and right now they look incredibly relieved. It's the mentors, James Hillman once said, who often see what the parent can't see: "The parent says, 'this is my child,' and that's fine for protecting it and feeding it and keeping it going. But every child has its own destiny. That destiny the mentor sees, takes care of, tries to teach."* And now for Frank, in this moment at least, the father finally sees it too.

After graduation I head for the Laundromat in Bicknell, wash my field clothes before heading out to Capitol Reef for a short hike, then back to the girls of Group 3. I'm stuffing clean underwear into the clothes drawer of the van when a guy in his sixties comes over, says he noticed my Montana plates, tells me he used to live there. After thirty seconds of small talk he launches into a tirade about the Park Service upping the fees for annual passes and how at the current rate of growth in ten years they'll cost a thousand bucks. "The government's screwing up everything," he assures me. He says he's a wildlife photographer, and when I make the mistake of mentioning I'd written a book on the Yellowstone wolves, it cranks him into a bitch session about how there was no excuse to spend a hundred million bucks on animals that no one will ever see anyway.

I can't say why this guy bugs me so much. After all, in the West, antigovernment diatribes are common as magpies on a roadkill. Maybe spending the last month elbow to elbow with kids who are locked in an epic struggle for personal control, for the wisdom and courage needed to own their lives, has left me

*James Hillman, interview, "The Best of Our Knowledge," National Public Radio, June 1977.

hypersensitive to anything that smacks of whining. "For God's sake," is what I want to say. "The sun's out. There's a restaurant full of hamburgers and french fries and pie fifty yards away from where we're standing, and a waitress named Debbie who used to wear a leather jacket and ride a Harley-Davidson who'll serve it up to you and make you laugh the whole time you're eating it. A few miles up the road are a thousand nooks and crannies in what may be the most beautiful slice of high desert on the face of this earth, where you could probably sniff out God himself if you were so moved, and here you are wasting time whining about the friggin' government." That's what I want to say.

CHAPTER TWELVE

WILDERNESS THERAPY ACCORDING TO
FRANK SINATRA

IT'S WELL AFTER dinner when Brad gathers his gear and pre-pares to walk out after a day with the boys, though not before calling a confab with staff at the edge of camp. "Listen," he whispers. "You've got to keep pushing. These guys are getting to where they can function out here pretty well, removed from things. But trust me, their parents are going to push their buttons five minutes after they see them. They'll spend two months thinking about getting back to their families, then want to blow them off once they get there. You need to push so they can learn to work through it." (This may be the only job on earth, I've heard instructors say, where when things are going really well, you know you're doing something wrong.)

I'm picking up on something big, a revelation of sorts, a shift in the boys' perceptions that's hard to imagine happening anywhere but out in the great wide open. Three weeks ago, say a big rain came along, the newcomers treated it like a personal slap in the face, as if the world were picking on them. This afternoon, though, when it starts raining and hailing like crazy, they don't necessarily like it, but they deal with it. I ask Shawn about it, and he says it happens all the time. "They start paying attention to what they're projecting onto their surroundings. The light goes on—you can see it. 'Maybe this doesn't mean I'm a shithead after all. Maybe it just means I'm getting rained on.' " He says with time it's pretty easy to make that kind of leap out here, to begin seeing things as just what they are, nothing more; there's the trees and the sky, it's dark and it's light. "It's a lot harder to build that kind of perspective at home with other people, because everyone is always telling you the meaning of things. There's all kinds of noise.

"Let's face it," Shawn says. "Some people are fine being told how to operate. Give them a recipe for success, they'll follow it and do just fine. But for a lot of teenagers it's more like, 'Bullshit—I'm going to win in spite of your recipe.' That's why what nature shows them is so powerful. The wilderness isn't locked into a power struggle with them, judging them, trying to shove something down their throats. It just is. No matter what happens out here, it's up to them to choose the meaning. That's an incredibly important thing to understand."

.

Then again, maybe these good days owe a little something to our having spent the last forty-eight hours at Johnson Pasture, a place so beautiful it couldn't help but soothe the sad, the angry, or the ravaged. The meadows are thick and green and every-where dappled with wildflowers. Warblers are trilling, brown creepers whistling up and down the scale, Clark's nutcrackers squawking like hard-smoking old women clearing their throats. Elk Creek makes a slow meander through the glades, braiding around tiny islands of willow and horsetail, finally gathering it-self and running on, sweet and cool, down the aspen-covered face of the mountain. The storms have passed, and the boys can hardly believe the plate of stars overhead. Kevin's eager to point out the constellations Jesse taught them; everyone oohs and aahs at the occasional meteor.

The next morning, after breakfast, we launch into curric-ulum, and even that seems matched to place. It's an English lesson of sorts, a discussion about the idea of life as a journey instead of a destination. Several boys say they're bummed by what they see as the American desire to root itself in other cul-tures, to turn them into smaller versions of ourselves. "Get 'em hooked on materialism, just like we are. Hey, it's good for busi-ness."

Jeff, on the other hand, a lean, muscular kid from Penn-sylvania—clever as can be and he knows it—says one of the big stumbling blocks in the road to seeing life as a journey is our obsession with perfection—that we can't really be in the mo-ment as long as we're comparing that moment to some perfect vision of accomplishment. "The way I see it," he explains, "ev-eryone is already perfect who's willing to learn and grow."

Over time the conversation evolves into a talk about the role of pain. Shawn, the instructor, talks about how in the most difficult period of his life, when his dad, grandma, and grandpa all died within a couple of years of one another, and then shortly afterward, when he was spinning out of control, stealing and lying, finally coming here to this program—even those times held certain opportunities, blessings. Here especially, he says, the struggle was real. "It was the kind of pain that forced me to grow."

Steve wanders up after finishing with some of the kids on their student-growth books, kneels down with us, smiles around the circle. "Guys, it's like that Sinatra song about New York," he says. "If you can make it here, you can make it anywhere. This is life under a microscope, and if you can manage two months in the wilderness, learn to deal with what comes up here, then no matter what hard times wait for you outside this place, you'll be able to handle them."

Staff, of course, can feel the tide turning for the better, and over breakfast they huddle up to figure out how to keep things going in the right direction, encourage the boys to keep building on their strengths, keep opening lines of communication. While the girls in this program are eager to enter into all manner of discussion about what's on their mind, what they're upset about, the boys seem more inclined to bicker about the smallest, most ridiculous things imaginable, prodding each other until emotions are running so high they finally overwhelm the fear and reluctance to be real. The girls push each other's buttons with nothing more than a look, a whisper, a smirk. The guys use sledgehammers.

After a lot of discussion, Steve suggests using some challenge activities—physical problem-solving games—something that will force the group to work together. Shawn not only agrees, but decides that if the boys succeed they'll get back the brown sugar Brad took away from them last week for pilfering food from one another. Brown sugar. Out here that's better than ten free CDs and a new pair of Nikes. As Jeff puts it, "It's gotten to the point where I miss food more than I miss my parents."

The first event of this multilateral Olympics, and by far the most powerful, is an old classic called "the electric fence." The "fence" is a rope tied between two trees, about six feet off the ground, with all the guys standing on one side. The task is straightforward: Get everyone over the fence without touching it; once you're over, you can't come back to the other side. For Group 4 the first decision is easy. With all the boy power assembled in one place, they hoist Kevin up and catapult him over the top of the rope, a 250-pound javelin hurtling through the trees. That done, a few more catapults, and things begin to get sticky.

Two trees and a dozen feet of rope and it all comes out. It's like watching theater, like reading myth, the strengths and weaknesses of the characters standing in such obvious relief, teenagers with designs that are in this moment as clear as when they were toddlers playing in day care, oblivious that the world was watching. Jeff's intelligence and sarcasm, Dale's anger and strength; Todd wanting to find solutions but uncertain whether his are any good, and the battle between Tom's eager genius and the sadness that won't leave him alone; Jim's sense of humor and his prattling on ad nauseam, hyperbossing, like the Energizer Bunny with its paw stuck in a light socket. And the tension, fully palpable, of that need to stop letting impulses run amok, to be a team, to trade the fast ride on a rocket full of urges for this slow, agonizing trip of giving and taking, trying to get something done.

Kevin, the big kid I picked up at the airport, who for weeks now has been a kind of fire hydrant for the group's wise guys, knocks us over this afternoon by announcing that he wants to transition to eagle. "I want to make my parents proud of me," he says matter-of-factly. "I also want that internal-frame pack." I'm skeptical, as are most of the staff. Not that Kevin hasn't made great strides. That blanket of goofy lethargy he's kept wrapped around him is definitely sloughing off. What's more, he's asking for help, both from staff as well as from the other guys. "I'm new at this leadership thing," he told the group a couple of days ago, referring to his being the only buffalo. "I don't know how to go about it, what to do. I've never been a leader of anything before." Still, it's a long trail from mere confessions to being eagle, from showing your underbelly now and then to having the personal integrity to inspire right action in the group.

One of the first requirements for eagles on their way to the sky involves calling a group to accept responsibility for past actions, and Kevin is at least willing to go that far. After dinner all of us huddle around a fire rich with the smell of burning Douglas fir, under a sky riddled with stars. Kevin sits cross-legged in a pile jacket, the black stocking cap that never comes off, day or night, pulled down to a point just above his eyebrows, absentmindedly plucking pebbles from the dirt, recounting a rather long and ambitious history of stealing. He seems properly contrite about it, never giving the slightest hint that he still sees these as heroic acts. But then Shawn asks the one question everyone sees coming—everyone, that is, but Kevin.

"So how's it going now? Have you been able to control the stealing out here?"

A long pause. From my place across the fire he seems to be wearing the face of someone standing on a high dive, trying to decide whether or not to jump. Finally, looking down into his lap, he starts to answer, so quiet and full of mumble that Shawn has to keep asking him to speak up.

"I've tried. I'm trying hard right now, but I don't always manage to succeed." He looks up, finds several other kids nodding, rounds up some nerve, and keeps going.

"It wasn't so much the stuff I took. I just liked the feeling I got when I was stealing. When I stole something for a little while there was this happiness, and it was so much better than what I had the rest of the time—this lonely depressed feeling. I felt guilty at first. But the drugs helped take that away. Pretty soon I'd stolen so much it was like picking your nose—just a bad habit that you don't even think about.

"I think there's something about this place," he says near the end of the group, looking around, staring out beyond the flicker of the flames into the dark woods. "It's okay to look at things you were pretty sure you didn't want to look at."

Kevin's willingness to come clean about stealing seems to have left everyone in the mood for confession. Next it's Dale's turn. Midafternoon we're walking together through a boulder field at ten thousand feet, and out of nowhere he starts telling me about all the stuff he's ripped off, saying how at the time he was doing it he always had plenty of money in his pocket. Stealing music and food, clothes and money, even books. "It's stupid," he growls, clenching his fists. "The last time was about two months before I got here. I won't ever do it again. My mom and my grandma drove me to this store to look for some shoes I really wanted. Grandma's really sick—I think she's dying; she was waiting out in the car for us. As we're walking out I see these

Rollerblade wheels in a basket by the counter so I just grab a handful and stick them in my pocket, and they bust me. We get back out to the car and Grandma finds out, and she gets this really terrible worried look on her face. She opens the door and gets out, says she has to go sit in the shade, rest for a minute, and it's so hard for her to walk, she can barely make it across the parking lot. It broke my heart.''

We take a break in a sun-washed meadow where you can look out some hundred miles to the east, across the red rock waves of Capitol Reef, past the gray-green shoulders of the Henrys, into that bleak, bright wash of desert. Dale and I sit for a while, not saying anything. Finally I ask about his family.

"My dad's okay, I guess. Stupid, though. When I was ten he was into drugs—mostly smoking a lot of pot. On weekends he'd have friends over, do hard stuff. I remember this like it was yesterday: He was out on the deck, totally stoned, and my mom walks out there. She tells him he'll have to make a choice—either give up drugs or leave. It was like my dad didn't really have to even think about it. He turned and looked right at her and he said, 'Fine, I'll leave.' That's what he did. And he never came back. It was the worst thing he could ever have done to us.''

I ask if he thinks his dad regrets it.

"All the time. He's got a great job, but he's lonely. All he does is work. When I got busted in school for dealing crack he freaked out. He pushed hard to send me here—says he doesn't want me to end up like him. I don't know, I still support him. I still love him. I mean he's my dad.

"What I do in life is based on what I want to do," he announces, suddenly full of cool, as if he'd shown too much. "I wanted to deal drugs, so I did it. I wanted to play baseball, so I did it.''

Then again, when Shawn calls us off the break, Dale shuffles over to the edge of the woods and hefts his survival pack onto his shoulders one more time. And it doesn't look at all like something he wants to do.

Two hours later in a hollow thick with pine, one final rest before going on to camp. A mile or so back Tom found a bow Kevin had dropped and declared it a ground score, his for the keeping. In retaliation Kevin grabs Tom's "possibles bag" (a canvas shoulder bag kids carry with them), calls it a ground score, and is refusing to give it back. The two of them are arguing like fish hawkers. Suddenly Shawn stands up and shushes them, pointing to a trail some fifty yards away where a group of boys from the adjudicated program are walking by. Big, tough-looking kids. Gang bangers and armed robbers. The players. Kevin and Tom quiet down right away and look on, wide-eyed, seemingly a bit fearful, though neither would ever admit it. In a couple of heartbeats they go from cocky to subdued, and they stay that way long after the other group has passed out of sight. As if that trail through the dark woods might be their trail; as if those sullen, dispirited looks might one day be their look as well.

CHAPTER THIRTEEN

THE NOT-SO-GREAT ESCAPE

THERE'S A CUSTOM of sorts around here that staff going into the field leaves bags of goodies in the car for those heading out. Most take a fairly health-conscious approach, buying bagels, maybe a little cream cheese, lots of orange juice. Not this week. This week we fall off the mountain with Cokes and Sprites and Doritos and sub sandwiches in hand—a collection of exactly the foods the kids talk about nearly every day. In truth I feel a bit off stuffing my face like this, equal parts guilt and contamination. Still, the leaving goes better this time. After unloading the car I head over to Wanda's with Steve for the usual rehash of the week, and then back to the house to help Dave plant garlic in the garden.

The next day I keep to myself, do some walking up the washes north of Bicknell, put some Dave Matthews and Robert Earl Keene on the stereo, try to get a little writing done, basically stay away from anyone but Dave, my trainer, who's been here plenty long enough to know the need to talk about things besides the kids up on that mountain. By the time we head off together for a late dinner in Torrey I'm beginning to feel refreshed, balanced, living in a larger frame again. The world continues to expand over nachos and flatbread pizza and Key lime pie. Conversations are all over the map: the struggle of the baby boomers to anchor themselves in community, speculations about native relationships to nature, tales of a former staffer who roams the West in an Airstream trailer, calling himself the Pilgrim. Dave talks of an old woman who used to come to this restaurant, would sit at your table and play bluegrass in exchange for food. We yak for hours, finally head for home around nine-thirty.

Another day or two of this, I'm saying to Dave on the drive back, and I'll be a new person. "You can't give to them," he answers back, "if you don't do a little giving to yourself." Two miles out of Bicknell, down a long straight run of highway ripping through the alfalfa, we spot the flashing red lights of a police car and headlights from several other vehicles parked along the ditch line. We go slow, figuring it to be the scene of an accident, somebody having nailed a deer or something, but as we get closer Dave notices that among the parked cars is one of our backup vehicles. Past that is the sheriff's car, and beside it a freaked-out-looking, brand-new twenty-two-year-old field instructor named Tony. Another pickup, and then, floodlit by headlights, three kids in the ditch, two of them huddled and crying to a woman hovering over them with her arms around their shoulders, the third slightly off to the side, lying on his back, staring into the headlights. Our kids. Runners.

We ease past the line of cars and pull over against the ditch, walk back to Tony, the new instructor. He stands there sucking air, looking utterly bedraggled—face smudged, hair tossed and sweaty. Dave, on the other hand, though his head must be spinning, comes across as perfectly calm, asking for a rundown of what happened.

"Group Six," Tony pants, "up at Spruce Lake. It's getting dark, Danielle and I are preparing dinner. These three rummage through Carrie's backpack, end up taking a Leatherman tool, our maps, some water—both the radios, too." At this point I expect Dave to flinch, given the stern warnings staff get at training about keeping equipment under watch at all times; but if he's torqued about it, he doesn't let it show.

"They take off hell-bent down Spruce Creek, making for the highway. I saw them when they were about three hundred yards off—took a few minutes to grab some water and clothes. Started out after them." The drop down Spruce Creek is rugged, incredibly steep. Tony says he lost them twice, ended up cutting their tracks, finally caught sight of them four miles down the mountain, at Bicknell Bottoms. Mustering what little strength he had left, he stumbled over to the first house he saw, tiptoed past a snarling dog, and as luck would have it ended up on the doorstep of the program's nurse, where he called the sheriff and backup. What he couldn't have known was that by then the boys had already been caught.

On the surface it might seem like the worst of luck to be a desperate kid trying to flag down a ride on Highway 24, weary as a plow mule but seemingly close to making the big break, and then have the first car by end up being Talmadge, who not only works for this program but is one of the best trackers in the West. Actually, bad luck doesn't begin to describe it. Staff here have lost count of the times Talmadge "had a feeling" things were going to happen on a particular night, headed over to a small trailer he keeps on Notom Bench, and then, for reasons that only God and Talmadge can imagine, started driving the highway and came across runners. Once or twice you could chalk up to coincidence. But it's happened a lot more than that.

With tears running down their faces, wiping their cheeks with dirty hands cut from sliding down the mountain, the boys struggle to tell their story. "We ran away for Scott's sake," Wayne says in a numb, weary voice, pointing with his head over to the kid lying on his back in the ditch. "His back was really bad and they kept making him walk. We ran to keep him safe, to get him out of that abuse."

It's a clever story, I suppose, but not all that clever. And certainly not unusual. For a lot of kids the first order of business during their initial week here is to write a letter home chronicling the myriad ways they're being abused. Actually, it's not a bad game plan, given that most parents have never even heard of wilderness therapy other than through a raft of stories about the tragedy of Aaron Bacon, who died at North Star. Years back—before the North Star incident—one of the more dynamic instructors decided he'd take the bull by the horns, get the whole "I'm being abused" stuff over with right at the start. One day during journaling he gave an assignment: Write a letter to your folks chronicling in as much detail as possible how we're torturing you. "I'd prefer you be original," he told them, "but if you have to, feel free to use some of my favorites: Tying you to trees with barbed wire, hanging you by your ears, stoning you for not finishing your dinner." And so they did. Had a pretty

good time with it, too. Unfortunately, the office worker at base
who was in touch with the parents every week—the woman
who was supposed to let the moms and dads know those letters
were coming—had just quit, so the word never got out. Pam
says she got calls at all hours for three days straight.

The boys are loaded up and taken over to the clinic, where
Scott gets a thorough examination by the doctor; she finds a
tiny muscle spasm in his shoulder, gives him a hug, and hands
the staff a supply of Motrin. Dan and Wayne sit hunched over
in the waiting room, looking sorry, helpless, scared. Meanwhile
Dave and I hurry back to the house, spend fifteen minutes loading our backpacks, then rush back to the clinic. "If I recall,"
Dave says to me, "wasn't it you who at lunch yesterday told me
and Tony that the one thing you hadn't gotten to see here was
a runner?"

"I'll be more careful what I ask for," I promise.

The plan is for Tony, Shawn from backup, Dave, and me
to hike the guys back to their camp tonight, a seven-mile, four-
hour trek up some three thousand feet of mountain. When we
find Tony again, looking freaked to the point of collapse, Dave
tells him that he understands what a terrible ordeal he's been
through, that he should feel free to "check out" for a few hours
during the hike up, try to collect himself. Tony clearly appre-
ciates it, though he looks a little surprised, maybe having expected some sort of tongue-lashing instead.

We park the cars at the trailhead, motors running and headlights on, and one by one, each of the three boys has to strip
and be searched for knives, drugs, whatever. Scott has his possibles bag with him, and Shawn sits on the ground with him in
the beams of the headlights and goes through his stuff: a handful
of .22 casings he found near one of the camps, a bubble pipe,

a crumpled copy of the curriculum, and a black-and-white fishing lure, with no hooks. Throughout all this Dave and Shawn are completely calm, friendly to the boys, even joking with them.

After being searched Dan sits cross-legged at the edge of the road, hunched over with his stocking cap pulled down over his eyes, his shoulders shaking with the crying. Back at the clinic he told Tony he doesn't feel safe out here any longer, that he may try to kill himself if he gets the chance. When everyone is dressed again and packed up we huddle with the boys in a circle on the ground, the air full of chill, the only light now coming from my headlamp. Dave tells them in the calmest of voices that we're going back up the mountain, and to Dan, gently, that he's being placed on suicide watch, because the most important thing we need to do right now is keep him safe.

I have to admit that when I first heard Dan had been talking suicide I thought maybe it was a ruse, anything to keep from being sent back to the wilderness. But in fact he seems genuinely relieved when Dave talks about putting him on watch— like a boy wanting nothing more than to be taken care of, someone to tell him it's going to be okay. Despite his young age, I'll discover later, Dan has been bludgeoned by all sorts of terrible events. Not long before he showed up here, his best friend's father took his son and Dan to the park, sat down with them, pulled out a gun, stuck the barrel in his mouth, and pulled the trigger. Two months later the friend tried to kill himself and failed; six months after that Dan's brother tried it and succeeded. The urge to run down a mountain in the dark in hopes of escaping the program is in some sense remarkable; personally I'm surprised he can still stand.

We form a hiking line, placing each boy with a staff person

in front of and behind him, switch on the headlamps, and head
up the mountain. It's half past midnight.

Unknown to us, the remaining staff of Group 6, Carrie and
Danielle, are at this moment also groping their way through the
darkness, on another trail, part of a six-mile round trip from their
campsite to Snow Lake, where they hope to find another group
and a radio. With them is Darrell, the one remaining student of
the group, his head probably on fire wondering whether his
fellow captives made it to freedom. Running, I've discovered,
especially among the boys, is a nearly irresistible fantasy in the
early weeks here, especially in summer, when you can gaze off
the high plateaus of Boulder Mountain and see what seems to
be the warm, welcome glow of Torrey and Bicknell and, even
more enticing, headlights coursing down the highway.

But there's no one at Snow Lake. Group 3 was there the
night before, but they're gone now, sleeping soundly on some
other part of the mountain. Dejected, Carrie and Danielle turn
around and start heading back up the path to their camp at
Spruce Lake. Then, to add colossal insult to injury, a mile short
of camp the bulb on their one headlamp blows out, leaving
them in deep woods, not even a wisp of moon, the trail completely swallowed up in darkness. Danielle makes several attempts to find the route, nose to the tree trunks looking for
blazes, feet feeling for that trodden path, staying in touch with
Carrie by frequent shouts, all to no avail. By one in the morning
they know their only choice is to stay put until first light. And
thus begins a four-hour huddle for warmth, sitting in the dirt in
a grove of Douglas fir, waiting for the flicker of dawn.

Our group, meanwhile, even with lights, isn't without challenges of its own. The first leg of the trail proves fairly easy to
follow—we lose it only once, at a stream crossing. The real

trouble comes a mile later, at a couple of rocky water pockets surrounded by lowland marsh. The spur trail we're trying to follow grows smaller and smaller, then breaks into braids, then disappears altogether in a choking wall of elderberry and rose and wax currant. It's not that we're lost, exactly—we've got maps and compasses to keep us heading generally in the right direction—but instead of a smooth, steady climb on a path, now we're bushwhacking across a long run of ravines. Roller-coastering, scrambling up one side across volcanic rocks and through white, ghostly looking stands of aspen, then down through brushy tangles of shrubs and saplings. Over and over. Every fifteen minutes or so staff breaks, pores over the maps in the beam of a headlamp, speculates on when we'll intersect another trail while the three boys drop to the ground and immediately fall asleep. Even when we do finally hit a worn path it's tough to say exactly which one it is, or where we are on it, and so we give another half hour to going up the trail and then back down again in the other direction, trying to get oriented.

I get the feeling the boys figure this crazy bushwhacking is some kind of hazing we've orchestrated, a punishment for their having run. There's no small amount of fear in their voices, city boys barely a week out of civilization, stumbling around the wilderness in the black of night, by all appearances lost. "What about your headlamp?" Wayne keeps asking me. "What if a bear sees that, and is attracted by it? What if he comes for us?" At one point a barred owl flushes from a tree not three feet from Wayne's head, struggles mightily to gain a branch in a nearby ponderosa, finally settles in, and sits there, watching us pass.

By the time we find ourselves on familiar ground it's four o'clock in the morning, and we're still a good forty-five minutes from camp. Shawn launches a trivia game—"Who was Kermit the Frog's nephew? On what two days are no major league sports played?"—as well as a few brain puzzlers, trying to keep the boys going. It works for awhile, but about a mile from camp Dan dives into the hillside beside the trail, pulls his stocking cap down over his face, and begs us to let him stay there and die. When we finally reach camp the guys head for their sleeping bags, which are right where they left them some nine hours and eleven rugged miles ago. Wayne collects everyone's shoes and pants, hands them over to Tony. "Take them," he says. "We don't care if we ever see them again." And with that he collapses in his bag and is out like a light.

Shawn and Dave aᵣ̇ clearly surprised no one's in camp, finally figure that staff must have taken off for Snow Lake to look for another group. Shawn heads off for the lake while Dave and I stay behind, try to get a little shut-eye with our ears glued to the radio. "Why aren't they here?" Dave says. "Or else down at base? The only answer is that they're lost, and I pray to God that's not it." An hour later, just past dawn, the rest of the group stumbles back, looking ragged, frazzled, worn down, and tuckered out. We try for a little sleep, get maybe an hour. Around nine Danielle rouses the boys and tells them to get a quick bite to eat because we're going to circle up.

Last night on the mountain, when staff was huddling over a map trying to figure out where the heck we were, Dave turned to me and said what sounded like the strangest thing: "This is the perfect thing for these guys. It's exactly what they needed." Personally I'm used to thinking that if a kid did something like this he was bound to end up pissing off a whole lot of people, and that in turn would lead to some serious punishment. But there hasn't been any of that here. There was the business of having to hike back up the mountain, of course, but that was really nothing more than a logical consequence: You left the field, so now we have to go back. The whole time—sitting in the ditch, at the clinic, going up the mountain—everyone was without rancor. Even Danielle and Carrie, who are clearly embarrassed, even hurt, feeling they can no longer trust these guys, don't seem to be all that angry.

I'm guessing that it's in the quiet of that general calm, the not having to crouch under threat of some kind of terrible punishment, that the boys are willing to make comments, draw conclusions about what they did. "I just wish it could be like it used to be," Wayne says to me, halfheartedly shoveling in a few spoonfuls of cold oats, munching on gorp, on the verge of tears.

"And how's that?"

"Sitting around the fire. Having fun. Being a group."

By the time we circle up, Group 6, which hasn't shown the slightest desire to look at their issues—the boys who one of the instructors said had nothing whatsoever going when it came to soft skills—are coming into the game. It's exactly what Dave was talking about when he said this was what these kids needed; a teachable moment, if you will. The trick now is to get them to relate what they did last night to how they've handled things at home. Wayne kicks things off, saying how when things get rough with his dad, his reaction is to run out of the house and not tell anyone where he's going—be gone for hours. Not surprisingly, he has huge trust issues with his parents. And now the same thing all over again, out here in the middle of nowhere.

Dan says more or less the same thing. But he also ventures a prediction about how his parents are going to react to his having run. "It was a spur-of-the-moment stupid mistake. But when I get home they'll treat me like a criminal." Danielle reminds him that there's a lot of time between now and then.

"You're out here for you, Dan, not them. Take advantage of it."

All three boys say they had a bad feeling about taking off, that they knew they were making a mistake before they were even down the first slope, still within a hundred yards from camp. "But I just kept running," Scott says. "I just put it out of my head and I kept running."

"Look, you guys were doing what you needed to do," says Carrie, a comment that leaves the guys looking confused. Seeing Dan here beside me, head hung, ready to collapse, I think it's probably a worthwhile point to make. She tells the boys it will take some serious effort on their part to build back the trust, but that doesn't mean she's going to treat them differently. She doesn't think less of them—only that she won't give them more rope than they can handle, more space than they can be responsible for. "Sometimes you have to take ten steps backward in order to move forward again," she tells them, saying that it would be ridiculous for her to expect them to come from a place of making poor choices at home and not make a few of them out here. Then, looking right at Dan. "The important thing is to not get stuck in your mistake. If you decide right now that you're an asshole, a jerk, then you're going to end up being that person. I want you to know that's not how I feel. When I tell you I can forgive you, I mean it."

The boys are asked to write out contracts, explaining in detail their commitment to this group—what kind of responsibility they're willing to take to make it work, how they intend to build back trust. Of course everyone will be sleeping in tight lines for a while; and Danielle especially, this being her first week as senior staff, will have one eye open through the night for a long time to come. She and Carrie and Tony are painfully aware of their own mistakes—having both radios in one place, not keeping staff packs in view at all times, and evidently Dave doesn't feel the need to hammer on it. This is one job, he's told me, where you have to learn to be hyperaware of doing things carefully. "I've got to get out of the field for a few months," Carrie says off to the side, shaking her head. "I've never, ever left a radio in my pack before. That was plain stupid."

If Carrie is frustrated, Danielle is hurting. Like so many other young staff I've met, she wants so much to trust. Trust, giving kids the benefit of the doubt, is what comes naturally to her. I get the sense she's thinking that to make this work she's going to have to say good-bye to a little of her kindness; and no matter how you look at it, that's a big price to pay. She too will have to be careful of burnout. Next week on her days off, camping in Grand Wash, she'll tell me about waking up in the middle of the night in a total frenzy, wondering where her kids are.

Shawn has been off the mountain for a good hour or more, having left as soon as he got word that Danielle and Carrie had returned; by now he's probably showered, stuffed a couple of Foodtown doughnuts in his face, and is back working his normal shift. Dave and I are supposed to be off today. Around noon we head down the mountain, end up doing yet another bushwhack, reach the parking lot in a hard rain. From there we head over to the Aquarius for dinner and a video rental, settle in at the house and play couch potatoes, drink Irish coffees, lose track of the movie plot because I can't stop talking about that crazy night.

CHAPTER FOURTEEN

DREAMING UP THE SUN

IF GENETIC MEMORY can be said to extend to something as nebulous as therapy, maybe I'm catching a whiff of it tonight. My last week with the girls of Group 3—in the high country, in a downpour. Kids and staff and Pam, the therapist, squeezing around the puddles, eyes flashing in the firelight, holding our breath against the smoke. It's as far from so-called normal conversation as you could get, and yet so much more familiar, so much more reassuring. Conversation as an old, sweet solace in the middle of a cold rain.

Melissa, a bright fifteen-year-old fresh in from New Jersey, is poking fun at the promotion video the company sends to parents. "There's this girl sitting on a rock, all smiles," she says.

"Clean, wearing street clothes—I mean, they made it look like some sort of field trip." At one point, for about five minutes, a hole opens in the clouds and a shaft of sunlight comes drilling through, amazing us all. "It's so holy!" Melissa exclaims, jumping up and running out into a nearby meadow for a better view.

The girls are eager to tell me about an eleven-mile trek they made yesterday over the Aquarius Plateau in rain and snow, some of them at various times thinking they were never ever going to make it. Susan especially fell into an old habit of feeling like a victim, claiming that her depression and her medication were keeping her from going on.

To be fair it was a tough, grueling piece of work—a lot more intense than most adults ever face. Besides, like many of us, Susan has for years been encouraged to embrace kind excuses over painful solutions. Be happy, we say over and over to our kids. Be comfortable. That's all we want for you. At the same time, of course, figure out how to muster whatever gut-level strength you need to stay off drugs, tell your truth, push through school when the world feels like it's falling apart around you.

Susan will tell me shortly after graduation that until she got into this program she assumed that the only way out of depression, to the extent that there is any way out, was medication. Other strategies that could at least help—exercise, social connections, building a relationship with her feelings—those things she never considered. Why would she? Drugs, instead of becoming one management tool, albeit an important one, became the only tool. "For a lot of doctors," says Alex, the senior instructor this week, "medication is the only resource they feel empowered to use. Not that those drugs aren't useful. But if that's all you've got, you can unwittingly enable kids in addictive behaviors. They end up feeling that the problem is beyond them, that they can't handle their emotions any other way. That leads to passivity—not just about the condition, but about a lot of things in life." Maybe Peter Kramer, author of *Listening to Prozac*, was right: There was a time not so long ago, he said, when we expected antidepressants simply to get rid of depression. Now we want them to take care of low self-esteem and fix personality problems, too.

Alex kept after Susan on that trek across the Boulder, encouraging her, prodding her through the sore feet and the cold and the exhaustion, and darned if she didn't make it. It's the first thing she tells me about when we get a chance to visit— going on for some thirty minutes about the horrors of it, all the while wearing the most terrific smile. Nine months from now she'll be sending me e-mail, still talking about that hike.

The only one who doesn't seem thrilled by the adventure is Brenda, who could walk the legs off a pack mule without breaking a sweat. For her it was no big deal, just another lousy day in the wilderness. Before dinner we huddle under the staff tarp while Brenda reads her mother's impact letter—that first piece of correspondence a kid gets from her family, one that's always read in group. Her mother says much the same thing most parents do—telling her how much she loves her, how disappointed she feels at the loss of the "good, energetic, kind girl you used to be." Brenda looks up at us with a stony face and announces that her mother is "not too bright." Fielding questions by the other girls, she tells us she began feeling depressed in seventh grade, about the time she started drinking heavily. According to her the drinking was just something she liked to do, and she could take it or leave it.

"I liked it best when I was all alone," she says, referring to that time when her mother's boyfriend was paralyzed in a car wreck, requiring such constant care that Brenda was able to run free without anyone having time for her. When the boyfriend grew too weary to carry on, and on that hot summer morning ended it all in her mother's bedroom with a gun to his head, it was the beginning of Mom coming back to her daughter, worrying about her, instead. As far as Brenda is concerned, she'd rather Mom would just go away.

That conversation may not sound like progress. But in truth it's a huge deal that Brenda is finally talking about the things that bother her—something she's never, ever done before—not here, and from what her mother says, not anywhere. The change, the staff tell me, started last week, on a terrible afternoon that left everyone gasping in the dirt. Like a lot of kids, one of the things Brenda has trouble with out here is staff change. Some have suggested she's close to having a borderline personality disorder, which could leave her inclined to see the current staff as good, or at least tolerable, and the incoming staff as pure evil. After last week's changeover she got so upset she began abusing the instructors, first verbally, calling Jonathan a "faggot bastard," then spitting, finally kicking and throwing rocks. And Brenda can throw rocks like a major league pitcher. Staff tried consequences of one kind or another, all to no avail.

"We finally put her on separates," Jonathan explains. "Danielle and I stayed with her while Jimmie and Laura hiked ahead with the rest of the group. We told her we were going to do everything possible to keep her safe, but that there would be boundaries." Another round of curses, and Brenda gets up, walks off, Danielle and Jonathan follow, try to coax her back. She starts punching them, violently kicking and clawing— Jonathan stops the story to show me the long, deep red scratch marks on his arms. At that point he and Danielle face the thing that no staff out here ever wants to face—the need to physically control a kid, bring her to the ground as gently as possible, subdue her, let her cool off. Even now, the telling of it leaves Jonathan shaking.

"It was the worst experience of my life," he says sadly. "All the while Danielle and I were trying to bring her to the ground I kept thinking of her brothers doing the same thing to her all those years—ganging up on her, taking her down, then raping her. This incredible struggle she was putting up, it must have gone on for twenty minutes, kicking Danielle off her legs and sending her flying through the air. And then a total giving up—silent, submissive. I get sick thinking about it." I search hard for some word of comfort, can say only that maybe it was good to the extent that this time, maybe the first time ever, somebody was physical without it coming to a horrible end, without it being a total violation.

After the takedown Brenda simply walked over to her gear, rolled up her pack, said she was ready to rejoin the group. The next day Alex and Elizabeth showed up to lead Brenda on a quest—an intense semisolo of sorts, lots of walking and talking, intended to knock loose a few bricks from the walls she's built inside. "For the first two days we walked and walked," Elizabeth recalls. "Bushwhacking, trudging through deep snow on the plateau. It never phased her." Then, on the third morning, she started talking, a little at first, and then more, opening up about the anger she feels toward her mother. When she came back to the group she was willing to be there. And that alone seems close to a miracle. "It's a perfect example," Alex tells me, "of us not really knowing what we did, or exactly why things worked out. A lot of times I'm in the dark about why a quest works. But there are plenty of times when it does."

Alex has told me over and over how these kids aren't problems to be fixed, but rather "people with gifts they haven't yet
realized." There's something these kids are missing, he likes to
point out, and it's also missing in the culture. "It's the realization
they matter. That their existence matters. Their impulses, their
words and conceptions and feelings—none of it's incidental to
who they are. None of it is there by accident."

I once overheard him saying that if these kids have anything in common with one another, it's an almost overwhelming
sensitivity to the world around them; that, and an incredible
knack for spotting bullshit. He sees those as gifts. And like most
gifts, they come with a lot of baggage. Curiously, while some of
the other staff I've worked with have fairly strong feelings about
what kinds of kids benefit from an experience like this and
which ones don't, Alex won't even play that game. "One kid
may come here, go through the program, and she's only ten feet
down the road. Maybe that'll be Brenda. Another comes in, and
she's already farther along at the beginning than where the other
kid ended. Granted, we screen against certain kinds of condi-
tions. But if you get here in the first place, and you stay here,
you're going to take something away from it."

Unlike most instructors, Alex didn't bring to this work an
unflappable passion for the out-of-doors. He didn't come here
from Outward Bound, or NOLS, or a rope course. He came from
corporate America, where he dressed up every morning and
drove to work at a computer firm in the big city, just like millions of other guys. After five years he grew sick of it, took a
deep breath and made a break, decided to come here, begin the
thing he felt most drawn to.

Alex says that when he first got here he tended to look at
the wilderness as a kind of extra, something incidental to the

job. Over time, though, he's come to see the genius of the setting, to know that what happens in the wilds probably couldn't
happen anywhere else. "Nature forces structure. Period. At
home you go for a glass of water, and if the faucet doesn't work
it's the plumber's fault. You get thirsty out here, you go find the
water on your own. You just can't displace responsibility. And
that makes a huge difference in a kid's ability to grow." He tells
me that if I don't believe it I should go visit an aftercare program. The difference between a kid who goes there straight
from home and one who goes there from the field, he assures
me, is night and day.

The Wawup Plateau is big, sweeping country, a grand toss of
paintbrush and grass and piñon and pronghorn, all of it laying
gentle on the eye, a childhood dream of summer made flesh.
Day after day off to the west above the Tushar Mountains, we
watch the June thunderstorms build out of thin air: blankets of
wool-colored clouds pushing through the afternoon across this
enormous sky, swelling with every mile as if they were taking
breath, finally loosing their cargo of rain right on top of us before drifting onward and downward, disappearing in the desert
like fog in the fingers of the sun. To the north rise Thousand
Lake Mountain and the Fish Lake Plateau, green as Canaan, full
of promise.

To a few of the girls, though, there is one creepy thing
about this place—the fact that a hard winter has killed a lot of
deer, leaving bones and hides scattered about. Heather, whose
imagination is forever in high gear, seems the most put out by
it, predicting the place will lead to terrible dreams, as if that
were something new. "We're sleeping on a killing ground," she

whispers to me, her voice full of intrigue. I find myself wishing we were back in the glory days of the southern Paiute—that we had in our company one of the celebrated Kaiparowits woman chiefs who could put her arm around Heather, tell her how the people are wedded to dreams—remind her that the danger is never in the dream itself, even a terrible one. The danger is only in the forgetting.

Heather's ADD behavior is a tiny fraction of what it was during her first week, when I was talking to her around the fire, making bagels. Back then it was hard for her to finish a single long sentence, let alone try to make fire or roll a survival pack, without throwing up her hands and walking off in a huff. These days she's cooking meals, conversing at length with staff, patiently helping one of the new girls work on the bow drill. It's nothing new—I've seen the same thing happen to a lot of these kids, drug addicts and nonusers alike. It leaves a lot of us wondering if ADD is a logical, even predictable loss of focus, clarity shredded by the noise and visual bedlam of modern life.

The night groups seem more real now. This evening we begin with Brenda, try to finish what we couldn't yesterday. No sooner do we get started when the wind kicks up out of nowhere, pelting us with scattered drops of cold rain, as if the gods had concluded that any story Brenda tells deserves a little extra drama. Alex starts out by having her read her mother's letter again. Unlike almost any other boy or girl I've seen, there's no pause, no catch in the throat in the reading of "I love you," no tears at the "I always thought we would be friends, would help each other through life. Now I don't even know you. I miss my little girl."

She tells us she likes living with her father better, even though he's strict, but that he doesn't seem to want to spend time with her anymore. Questioning by Nancy, the girl who's been struggling with bulimia, leads her to admit that her dad used to beat her, "but not so much any more. He'd hit me if, like, he caught me smoking in his house, but now sometimes I smoke there when he's out and he doesn't even say anything about it. I know he can smell it." And in that statement is the first real sadness I've heard in her voice, as if the beating was from a time when he was at least in her life, when he cared enough to have her there. And now there isn't even that.

Alex brings up the point to Brenda that she doesn't seem to accept compliments about how well she does things. "I can do things if I want to," she tells him. "I just don't want to." Kate, the instructor from Vermont, doesn't buy it. "It sounds to me like you're saying you can do a lot, but not really do anything well. Someone has told you you're not good at things, that you're not good enough as a person. Part of what we're doing here is to help you reverse that." Brenda nods, her head down, and in the dark and with the wind blowing her hair I can't tell, but for a minute I wonder if she's crying. Alex asks the rest of us to tell Brenda whenever we see her doing something well, even though she might not accept it.

There are poems tonight. Hard-edged stuff, full of anger. Melissa, from New Jersey, reads a couple she just finished. The first is thick with sarcasm, talking about the lack of real values in society: "It's all about what plastic is and never who's within." And how "the only happiness is a synthetic smile, with lies and scams and media and anorexic Barbie dolls":

> Fucking around with your boss just to keep your job,
> being told you can't do shit by plastic surgeon Bob;

marry men with lotsa cash just to take a trip,
getting laser surgery because you got a nick . . .

Her second one is even less kind, raging against the abuse
she's suffered from the males in her life. She talks quietly, but
often, about the boys who will say anything to get her into bed.
Also about unsettling feelings toward her father, who as of late
has been encouraging her to take care of him in unfitting ways,
do things like trim his hair and cut his fingernails, leaving her
feeling "like a mistress." This one she calls simply, "My Boys":

> You asshole,
> you son of a bitch (actually, I liked your mom)
> every motherfuckin' one of you.
> You all took me (in more than one way)
> and you told me so much bullshit
> (actually everything you say is bullshit)
> and you twisted and fucked with my mind
> to make me believe you cared.
> Then you leave.
> Well listen, asshole,
> I USED YOU TOO.
> So fuck you.
>
> Love,
>
> Melissa

There's also talk tonight of ritual, ceremony. Nancy swears
she's going to keep doing solos after she gets home, and several
of the rest of the girls, including Susan, agree. Melissa hasn't
been here long enough to have a strong sense of such activity,
but tells about making rituals of her own. Like when her boyfriend broke up with her last winter and she went home, locked
her bedroom door, and cut off all her hair.

Just as we're about to break for the night, Beth, the meekest of all the girls, finds her voice for the first time, saying how difficult it is for her to say what she wants to say, that she tends to sit on her feelings, lets them build up until they come out in fits of rage. "I handle things by holding them in. And then I don't handle them at all. That's when drugs look best." I notice the other girls nodding their heads.

"When I was in the suicide ward, we used to have a punching bag—you know, so we could get out our anger. I loved it. Then they took it away. They told us it wasn't appropriate to respond to anger by being physical. But they didn't give us anything else. For me the talking won't come until the anger goes down."

Something about all this is hitting home with Kate as well. When the girls finish sharing she leans toward the flames, looks each girl in the face. She's sitting right beside me, and in the firelight I can see tears slipping down her face. "Please listen to me," she says, with an intensity so out of character for the Kate we've come to know that it leaves us all holding our breath. She tells of struggling with similar issues her whole life, using alcohol to blunt the pain, just like her dad did, doing anything she could to cover up that voice. "Take responsibility for your own well-being," she tells them. "Say what you need to say. Don't hide behind the blaming."

Watching Kate reeling from her own wounds reminds me of something Alex told me two months ago, when he first heard I was writing this book. A remark that at the time I didn't understand. "I'm no writer," he said. "But if I were telling a story about this place, there'd be a lot of times when it would be pretty unclear whether the voice was coming from a student, or from the staff."

Having endured several days of rain and cold, when the

girls ask for a story before bed I decide to go with "The Birth
of the Sun," from Australia. It's a tale about how long ago two
large birds of that country, the emu and the brolga, were fighting with each other, trading insults about how wonderful their
own children were and how god-awful ugly were the kids of
the other. Finally the emu gets so upset she hurries over and
swipes one of the brolga's eggs with her bill, and with a great
heave tosses it into the heavens, where it lands in a massive pile
of sticks gathered by the sky people, setting it afire.

*Now up until this time there had been no light on
earth, and when the sky people gazed down to see how
beautiful the place was, shimmering in the firelight, they
decided to light a fire every day. It starts out weak, in the
morning, when the burn is just starting, but by midday
it swells into a great bonfire. This burns down during the
afternoon, and finally goes out, giving way to night.*

*The only problem was that the sky people depended on
sighting the morning star to know when to light the fire,
and on cloudy days that didn't work at all. So they asked
for help from the kookaburra bird. Every dawn, cloudy
or clear, that bird lets out a pealing, rollicking laugh,
letting the sky people know the time has come to touch
off the woodpile and light the world.*

I tell the girls I hope the story helps them dream up the
sun. For good measure, Kate leads us in a rousing chorus of
kookaburra calls.

My last night in the field, and it's rich. Sometime around
one in the morning an elk herd stumbles across our camp, takes
a whiff and grunts loudly, then starts running lickety-split across

the talus slope right above us, a great thunder of hooves and rocks crashing down the mountain. A little later an entire chorus of coyotes lets loose—the first full-on pack singing I've heard in a long time.

Not all is bliss, though. Susan, now just days from gradua-tion, has a terrifying dream. She's here on the Wawup Plateau, packing up a few things for what she assumes is a routine trip out of the field for a psychiatric evaluation. In the distance she spots what look to be a couple of forest rangers, standing near a bus—she waves, they wave back, she walks over and gets on, figuring it's going to town. But once on board, once the doors are closed and the bus is rolling down the mountain, to her horror she real-izes it's going to "a really terrible mental hospital, for really crazy people." She panics, starts breathing hard, trying to figure a way off the bus, wakes up mumbling in a pool of sweat.

Evidently the kookaburra calls worked, because the next morning is brilliant, not a cloud in sight. Sweet yellow light is falling on the pockets of aspen around our camp, lighting the clematis and the paintbrush blooms, steaming the ground until it's thick with the smell of wet sage, pulling nearly every girl, each in her own time, slightly off to herself, head turned to the sky. Melissa is way into it, taking deep breaths, looking like someone reborn. "Another holy day!" she says to me. "Hey, did you know that God is the man in the moon?"

We begin the day with curriculum, then Kate helps the girls finish some art projects they started yesterday, using brushes made from yucca stems, the fibrous ends pounded and fuzzed into bristles. As with the boys, it's interesting how many of them say their work is "stupid," or "not any good," when in fact much of it is really quite beautiful. Their comments seem to speak to a deeper problem, this inability to build a relationship to their creativity, the dark and the light of it, the thing that makes them truly unique in all the world. I share an old piece of advice for writers—about how, instead of trying to think things up, it helps to instead simply write things down—as if you were a scribe, tapping into passions and stories that are already out there, and in the process, lifting from your shoulders the need to create something perfect out of nothing. It strikes a chord for some, as does a comment Jonathan makes about dance, about how things really start happening for him during a performance at the point he stops doing, and just starts being. It's the perfection thing, several of the girls agree, that always trips them. "There are so many things in my life," Melissa tells us, "where it feels like I'm just not good enough."

We break around noon to play a few games. Nancy, feeling sorry for me, finally tells me the secret of "Billy Williams" and "stick dance," neither of which I've ever figured out. Brenda, who's actually enjoying herself, comes up with the solutions to both of them with no help at all.

And so wind down my last precious hours in the field. A final round of the stuff of life—a few smiles, a little understanding, the comfort held in the voices of your friends. I'll miss all of it. The smell of wet grass mingled with hints of sweat and bean farts, the snoring, Heather holding spitting contests along the road. I'll miss carving wooden spoons, playing Ali Baba around the fire, the sitters, and the runners. The transition rituals and the good-bye groups, the bow-drill fires, and the strange, superstitious chant of "I hate white rabbits" the girls use to try to drive campfire smoke out of their faces. The wind and the rain, the dust, and Melissa, out there even now, smiling up into that blue, blue sky.

CHAPTER FIFTEEN

REUNION

A DAY OFF before helping out with graduation. The final act of passage not just for me, but for Kevin and Susan and Nancy, as well as for Keith, whom I haven't seen since picking him up at the airport, listening to him in the back of the Suburban, asking whether the speakers had been torn out by some kid who went crazy; and later that same day, standing beside him at base as he huddled in the supply room, being strip-searched—wanting to throw a blanket around him, toss him in my van, and drive him home.

The fields around Loa lie sweet and green under the June sun, pampered by the spray of enormous sprinklers running day and night. A few of the watering systems are slightly misplaced, pumping water in a hard splatter across the windshields of the tourist cars roaring up Highway 24, making for Capitol Reef. The fencelines are on fire with the orange blossoms of a thousand globe mallow, broken here and there by lavender runs of thistle. On the domestic side, in the two weeks since I headed up the mountain, Dave's garden has found its heart; we eat radishes and spinach and onions, sometimes raw, sometimes for dinner, great, steaming skillets of them on the electric range.

I grab a few radishes and a patio chair, carry them up to the roof and sit for an hour, soaking up the sun. To the south is a clear view of the Boulder, free at last of all signs of snow. In April it was just a beautiful mountain. Now it seems so much more—staging ground for forty-eight kids, all of whom this very minute are either hiking or pushing carts, the newcomers cursing their fate, while the ten about to graduate are locked in heartfelt good-bye groups. Some of those, including Susan and Nancy, are crying over having to say farewell to what they say is the only real taste of community they've ever had.

Last night there was a concert at the Roost Bookstore in Torrey, bluegrass with the Foggy Notion Boys, from Portland. Afterward several of the field staff sat around for a couple hours and jammed with the band. Alex had a mean guitar going, leading the pack on "Train Train" and "Angel from Montgomery," while Kate took care of the spoons and Greg, the banjo. Around eleven o'clock Jonathan showed up with his Australian didgeridoo. At the end we all sang "Amazing Grace." The kids would have liked that.

This morning I run into a couple of staff at the Aquarius, Greg and Ryan, about to head off to do a sweat in an old lodge at Grouse Creek, and they ask if I'd like to come along. When I get there around three o'clock no one's around, so I spend some

time watering my memories of this exact spot: The three days
I spent last fall hanging out with a coed group, watching a couple of boys, newcomers, looking awestruck by two strong, remarkable girl eagles. And more recently, with Brenda on suicide
watch, then with Group 4, playing tag with a dodgeball one of
them found along the road, stumbling through the sage and cutting my legs and laughing like I haven't laughed for a very long
time. The lupine is tall now, in full flower, and the bitterbrush
is just starting to show blooms. The wild roses have faded, their
sweet scent gone for another year, replaced by the dry, hot
smell of ponderosa.

After waiting a while longer, reading, writing, sitting in the
sun, by five I figure Greg and Ryan aren't going to make it after
all and decide to carry on myself. I dig the stones out of the pit
at the center of a lodge that looks something like a root cellar,
carry them up to the fire ring, gather wood from across the
creek, fill the pouring jug, pull out my bow-drill set, and build
a fire, begin heating the stones. The thought of rolling red-hot
rocks down the path from the fire pit to the lodge makes me
nervous about the chance of forest fire, so while the stones are
cooking I get down on my knees and clear away pine needles
with my hands, scraping the path down to bare dirt. Half buried
near the door of the lodge is a crumpled, handwritten note,
which I stuff into the pocket of my shorts. A light rain begins
to fall.

Then the waiting for the rocks to heat, a good couple of
hours. I stroll the grounds, dust off some more memories, head
into a nearby field to pick some sprigs of sage for the sweat. On
the way back to the fire I look up to see a rainbow in the east,
glowing against pearl-colored clouds. When the stones are
ready, instead of rolling them I end up using a large flat rock

like a platter, carrying them one by one back down the hill and then pushing them through the door and into the pit. When the last rock is in I take off my clothes, wiggle through the tiny opening, pull the tarp door closed behind me. I close my eyes in the darkness, hum a quiet song I've never heard before.

Though I've done several sweats with Native Americans, I'm not a part of that culture and never will be, and it seems more than a little disingenuous to copy what I've seen of their tradition. Still, there's something altogether familiar about this sitting through round after round of steam, the sweat rolling out and the smell of sage filling the darkness, much as there's something familiar in the motion and the scent of a bow-drill fire.

Tomorrow, as luck would have it, I'll meet up with the graduating students not far from here and at the suggestion of an instructor named Jason, eight of us—including Nancy, Kevin, and Keith—will end up huddled together in this same lodge. Maybe it's because of the gravity of finding themselves poised on the edge of leaving, but I'll be struck by the fact that not a single kid will fail to treat the experience with reverence. After the first pour of water, at Jason's request I'll tell them the African story of the bird who laid her eggs on the plain—the one I told Carla the day she made eagle. I'll say again how some consider that story a touchstone for knowing how to treat the children of our higher natures—our ideas, our inspirations, and our urges to create—how there are times when we have to carry those things to new surroundings, plant them in new places, let them take root among new relationships.

Jason will begin each of three rounds of steam with an invitation to voice thoughts and prayers: in the first round, a hope for someone else; in the second, for ourselves; and in the third, for the future. One kid will ask that her parents come to see her as she is, instead of how she once was. Another will send good wishes to a friend back home, a boy in a gang who's in great danger. Still another will ask blessings for his father, a homeless man, a drug addict wandering the streets of Seattle— praying that one day he'll be able to take him in and care for him.

In a sweat lodge, much as in dreams, time melts, loses its handles. By the time I crawl out tonight and jump into Grouse Creek, nearly two hours have passed. There's a group of adjudicated kids from the AYA program about a half mile down the road, at the grad site; to avoid disturbing them I head back to the van cross-country, through the woods, thinking of absolutely nothing but the feel of my feet touching down on earth, scuffing against logs, wading through the stream. The rain has stopped, and stars are beginning to peek out from behind a tattered veil of clouds. My bare legs brush against the wet leaves of the rose and the lupine, and there are times when it feels like I'm gulping at the smell of willow and pine.

Right as I'm about to drive off I remember the crumpled note I found at the door of the sweat lodge, pull it out of my pocket, give it a look under the interior light. It's a smattering of free verse, almost certainly from one of the students in this program, or AYA, both of which use this area nearly every week. One more kid, trying to imagine life after the wilderness.

> Rollin' round da hood with my homies sippin' on a 40,
> smokin' on blunt,
> thinkin' 'bout the old days,
> talkin' 'bout the new day.
> Where we gonna be, how we gonna be, who we
> gonna be.

In 1982 a professor of ethnology working in Utah came across a direct descendent of the Paiute—an old man, eighty, maybe ninety years old. The professor spent several hours with him, asking what he remembered of the beliefs, the visions of his people. "Life for the Paiute is very hard," the old man said at the outset. "We suffer a lot. But I think in our hearts we are happier than the whites. We are happy because we know who we are."

While it may prove to be the most fleeting of feelings, the ten teenagers coming out of the wilderness today have had a chance not just to glimpse who they are, but in one or two quiet moments in the middle of nowhere, to celebrate it—at the edge of a desert wash, in the shade of a juniper, under the white arms of the aspen. Ask them in this moment and they'd probably say Ed Abbey was right—that we need to "appeal to the Indian, to the Robin Hood, to the primordial in every woman, every man—all who are still emotionally alive."

In the end, of course, some will turn away from all this, hide from the power of a new identity in drugs or possessions, replay the ancient myths of a sleeping youth who chooses to slumber rather than dance with the uncertainties of a new self. Others will use it—maybe tomorrow, maybe not for years—but with no less intention, no less sacred feeling than Tecumseh had for his *pawawka,* clasping it in his hand, leaning on it through that long, cold night before the dawn of manhood.

At last comes the morning of the run-in. Yesterday evening parents and siblings met in Loa to hear Brad talk about what their sons and daughters have been going through; again, most of them were dancing between the hope of a good reunion and

fear that things will be exactly as they were when Johnny or
Suzy left home two months ago. "We could see the changes
over time, in the letters he was writing," Keith's father tells me
this morning. "So we're hopeful. To tell the truth I'm so excited
I couldn't sleep."

Before we head out, Lavoy has his usual meeting with the
families, supposedly to tell them about the curriculum their kids
have been working on in the past two months, but as always,
thrilling them by spinning stories—on this day, tales about fire
and biology, with the beginnings of the universe tossed in for
good measure. Near the end of the session he talks about how
the vast majority of life on earth has evolved to propagate by
sexual reproduction. "And that kind of reproduction encourages
variety," he tells them, giving all sorts of examples, building a
road for them to think about their kids in a new way. "Nature
loves uniqueness," he says, and that makes them smile.

By noon we're out at the grad site, all set for the run-in,
the parents yelling into the hand-held radio a chorus of "Are you
ready!?," the kids shouting back, and finally, the scream of, "On
your mark, get ready, go." And then the long ten to fifteen
minutes of waiting for them to run the mile and a half down
that dirt road along Grouse Creek, many with tears on their
cheeks, stumbling across the finish line into the arms of moms
and dads and brothers and sisters. Even though I saw Keith at
the sweat yesterday, I'm still astonished by the change in him.
Not just a stronger, more muscled appearance, but the way he
carries himself, head up and shoulders back, looking whoever
he's talking to right in the face. He is an eagle. His parents, as
well as those of Susan, Nancy, and even Kevin, seem to be in a
mild state of shock, backing off from their hugs now and then
to run their eyes up and down their kids, laughing in disbelief

at how different they look from when they last saw them.

There's a different energy in this grad than in the one with Kristine and Sara and Frank. Even Nancy, who's certainly unsettled about seeing her father, seems for the moment willing to acknowledge that it's good for all of them to be together again—her dad, her mom, two older sisters, and an older brother. More amazing still, later in the afternoon every single parent shows a willingness to do the feelings checks and the sharing circles and the trust activities, at least make an attempt to overcome their self-consciousness for the sake of a place and a process that has left unmistakable footprints in the lives of their children.

By five-thirty the families are collecting their gear and being led off by their kids to their solo sites. Pam and the other therapists will visit each of the families they've been working with, one at a time, talking with them, offering exercises to help them stitch their lives back together against the inevitable resurfacing of old hurts, issues that haven't gone away. With their permission, I go along. Our first stop is Nancy, and walking into her camp I actually catch myself holding my breath.

Maybe it's the setting. That, and the fact that after two months apart everyone's emotions are running close to the surface, ready to either blossom or ignite. Still, I'm amazed at the power behind a simple, tried-and-true therapy tool Pam launches, called the family sculpture. The idea is for the student to create a living sculpture, placing her parents and siblings in various postures and positions to represent the dynamics of what was going on in the family when she left home, talking it through, explaining the meaning behind the placements she chooses. After this, she rearranges them to represent how she'd like things to be in the future.

It's round one—the one about how things used to be—

that's prone to explosion. Last fall I watched a divorced couple at graduation going through this, their daughter placing Dad in the middle with the kids, shoulders bent and head hung down, while Mom was out at the edge of the woods with her back turned to the family. Suddenly the mother broke down, seemed to forget her kid was even there, began railing against her ex-husband, cursing him. For whatever reason, there's an intense link between those body positions and highly charged memories, a rush that can kick down the door to things long forgotten, setting free a raft of anger and grief and regret. It's not a game for the faint-hearted.

And now Nancy, making a sculpture of her own. She stands her mom and dad and two sisters in the middle, and her brother, whom she says she really hasn't seen much of in recent years, on the outside, looking in. Her mom she places on her knees gazing up at her dad, who looms over her with his arms up in a muscle-man pose, looking stern. Her sisters are placed around her mother, as if trying to either comfort or protect her. As for Nancy, she's off to the side, halfway between her brother and the rest of the family—a no-man's land, not really a part of anyone's life.

And that's when Dad goes off. Nancy tries to talk to him, but he's way too upset to keep the reins on the format, especially the reflective listening part. Pam tries to bring him back, and he takes a potshot at her as well. Nancy suddenly gets a truly terrified look on her face, runs back to the road and disappears into the darkening woods. We wait for her while Pam tries to calm the family, and when she doesn't come back, one of her sisters and I go after her. We find her lying on her stomach in a patch of grass in the aspen trees, sobbing. She says she's too afraid to go back, that she doesn't know what her dad might do. That it's not safe. It's then that it finally sinks in for me—all the comments by the instructors and therapists about the need to push buttons out here in the wild, provoke, because no matter what kind of stressors a kid faces out here in the wilderness, no matter how many carts you push up the hill or rainstorms you curse or bows you bust in half because they won't make fire, it will be nothing compared to the power held in a couple of hours spent with family.

We talk to Nancy for a good ten minutes, remind her of the strength she's forged out here in the past two months, the solid center she has that no one—not even her father—can take away. Finally she agrees to go back, but with great reluctance, looking as though she's shuffling off to a beating. For a while she and Dad spar back and forth, him getting angry and pausing, checking himself, her retreating, cowering, then finally, the two of them talking again.

And then something incredible happens. In a flash of alarm that you can clearly see washing across his face, Nancy's father understands for the first time that his daughter is terrified of him. And that's not something he ever considered. The anger that was flaring a second ago drains away, turns to tears. He sits down, asks her to sit beside him, tells her that whatever he's done to set up that feeling, he is terribly sorry. He asks her forgiveness. He says he loves her. He explains that he grew up in a family where chaos was the norm, where everyone yelled all the time. Also, that in the business world being aggressive was how he kept things going. It was a mistake, he says, to bring that behavior into the house, and he's sorry he treated his family that way.

It opens up the floodgates for everyone to talk, to support Nancy, but also to bring up some of her manipulation, her being out of control—things she needs to work on. Twice she backs off, shuts down, starts to walk away. In the two months we spent with her, none of us ever saw that reaction, not once; yet from what her sisters are saying, it's standard stuff. Pam calls her on it, says she has to have the willingness, the courage to listen, just like she expects her family to do. Later Pam will tell us how she wishes she'd known about the shutting down, that she would have tried to prompt it out in the field, help her learn to recognize it, deal with it. Yet another example of a button that only the family can push.

On it goes. Nancy tells her oldest sister that she always wanted to be her, that she's spent her whole life putting on masks that made her look more like Rhonda, whom she thought the family liked better. "I've put on so many masks, for so long, I don't know who I am anymore." Through it all, especially in the worst of it, when it seems the whole family is in meltdown, the three women step back and look up through the branches of these magnificent aspen trees, almost as if they were breathing in the woods, calming themselves with the rustle of the leaves.

It's two and a half hours later when we finally leave them to their fire and their dinner. Before we go, Nancy's brother, who is a high-level manager, thanks Pam profusely, as if he's had a revelation. "I've never heard, never seen that kind of communication," he says. "I've been in so many relationships where I've just walked away."

Susan's sculpture, thankfully, is a lot easier to work through, though her dad—an accountant from the Midwest—has never done anything like this and is painfully uncomfortable. To his credit he keeps trying, keeps working at it, finally musters the courage to tell Susan he loves her, that her illness has never been a burden, as she often implies. Toward the end Susan's mother makes a remarkable comment. She says that in the past two months she's come to understand that she can't fix Susan's depression, can't make it go away, no matter how much she wants to. And more, that it's not her job to make it go away. Not her duty to make sure everyone in the family is always happy, without turmoil in their lives. It's a comment that people who come through graduation, especially mothers, end up making fairly often. And it never fails to leave the therapists relieved.

"It's a shame," Pam tells us back at camp, sitting around the fire. "We only get to work with the whole family such a short time. It'd be so exciting to keep going! Kids ask me all the time, don't you have a program that adults could come to? Don't I wish."

"The thing is," offers Jonathan, only half joking. "You'd need legal custody, because once the going got tough, half the adults would just split."

The moon hangs full tonight, lending plushy light to the sage and the ponderosa, not dropping over the western horizon until dawn begins to break in the east. Another cloudless day, calm, summer full on and, as far as we can tell, planning to go forever. One by one the families stumble out of the woods back to the grad site. Some tell us they went to bed early, exhausted, while others stayed up through the night, talking. A couple of the corporate fathers surprise me with their careless, somewhat disheveled look—in part, no doubt, thanks to the comfort of reunion, in part because of nothing more than the feel of sun on their faces and the smell of pancakes on the griddle. It's like some cherished but forgotten way of life has found them again.

Their kids cast furtive, sidelong glances at them, surprised not only that they're here but that they're present. "We get so many absentee, workaholic parents," a senior staff told me once. "Smart, competent people who know in the back of their minds that they need to be more involved with their kids, their families. But often it's like their own addictions, their habits of work and career, are just too much to overcome." At least there's this one good morning, I'm thinking. Mr. Executive, sitting on a stump by the fire with a paper plate full of pancakes, in need of a shave, syrup on his sweatshirt, his free arm around his son's shoulder.

The last ritual of the day, and the end of the wilderness program, is a ceremony called the Heartstick. Everyone (some forty of us in all) is sitting in a circle in a grassy meadow. A rock heated in the morning fire is at the center, and one by one the ten graduates place a sprig of green sage on top of it; the sage smolders there, and pungent wisps of smoke from the burn drift past our noses for a good hour.

The centerpiece of the Heartstick ceremony is an inch-thick, two- to three-foot-long tree branch, whittled by the students and sometimes carved with fanciful designs, deeply notched every few inches into clear segments, one for each graduate. The Heartstick is passed around the circle, and whoever holds it has the chance to speak about whatever seems important in that moment. It is one of the oldest communication rituals known to humankind.

Jason has asked me to tell a story before we begin, so I offer one from the Iroquois, the tale of the healing waters. It begins long ago, when a deep, fierce winter lay heavy on the forests of the Northeast.

In the midst of their struggle to stay alive the people were struck by a terrible illness, a plague that threatened to destroy the entire Iroquois nation. Nekumonta watched his relatives die, one after another. His sister and his brother. His father. One bitter morning he woke to find his wife with the sickness, and it was too much. He gathered his courage and walked off into the dark heart of the forest, determined to find where the creator Manitou had placed his healing herbs.

For three days and nights he wandered through the deep snow, sometimes on his hands and knees, asking the help of every animal he came across—the bear, the moose, the deer. But all just looked away, saddened by the hopelessness of the task. On the third night Nekumonta tripped and fell, and there he lay, too exhausted to get up again. In the dark of that long night the creatures of the forest gathered around him, watched over him. They knew him to be a sympathetic man, a compassionate hunter, a lover of the flowers and the trees. And in the darkest part of that night they sang out in pity, calling out to Manitou for help. And Manitou heard.

As Nekumonta lay sleeping, Manitou sent a messenger with a dream. In the dream his wife was singing a beautiful song that sounded like running water; soon that image melted away, replaced by the vision of a spring. The spring called to Nekumonta, telling him that in those waters he would find the promise of new life.

He awoke and looked all around him, but saw no water. Then he cocked his head, heard a faint trickle. It seemed to be directly under his feet. With flint and stones and the branches of trees he dug and scraped at the fro-

zen earth, hour after hour, until finally he reached the
sacred spring. He bathed himself, and remarkably, was
immediately strong again. Giving thanks, he fashioned a
jar of clay, filled it with the water, and headed back to
his village as fast as he could run. He gave his people
directions to the spring, and then hurried off to his wife.
Some of the precious liquid he poured between her lips;
the rest he rubbed on her brow and hands, and she fell
into a peaceful sleep. When she awoke later that after-
noon, the fever was gone. From that time on, Nekumonta
was known as the chief of the healing waters.

It occurs to me, I tell the people of our circle, that over
the past two months we too—students, parents, siblings—have
been on healing journeys of our own. Not searching for sacred
water, but searching for truth. And while it may seem that we
only glimpsed little pieces of it, even a few drops may have the
power to change our lives. The time has come this morning for
taking the truth to the people—just as the hero Nekumonta did,
giving water to his wife, his tribe. It's time to bring those truths
out in the open, to place them in this Heartstick circle and make
them real. With that Jason passes the Heartstick to his right, and
the parents, the brothers and sisters, the students, whoever
wants to, begin to speak, around and around again until there's
nothing left to say.

It goes first to Richard's father, a car dealer from Dallas,
who tells us that we're about to go to a dirtier, messier place
than this. "Our lives at home are filled with so many loose
ends," he says. "So many distractions. But we need to remember
that this is all the same world. That what we carry with us right
here, right now, we can carry there, too."

Nancy's father is on the verge of tears, and when the Heartstick reaches him he turns to his daughter, promises again that he'll do his best to communicate with her, then looks at his entire family, says he'll try to make life better for all of them. Her brother still seems amazed by the significance of what's happened to him in his short time here. He thanks everyone again for teaching him how to communicate—tells us he'll never forget it.

Susan's father, to my surprise, overcomes his shyness and finds the voice to tell Susan he loves her, out loud, in front of all these people. Her mother, on the other hand, closes her eyes, takes a deep breath, holds tight to the Heartstick. "I'm thanking God—not just for the staff and this program. But for this place. I suspect a lot of what happened here is thanks to the beauty and power of this place. Over the last day I've discovered that we're a strong family, a strong unit. It took coming here for me to know that, away from the familiar things I thought were so important to my life."

In one of the last rounds, Jason, the instructor, clutches the Heartstick in his hands and looks around the circle. "These are your kids," he says to the parents, his voice calm but serious, looking each one of them in the eyes. "Now you have the opportunity to help things get better, to talk things out. You need to take this opportunity very seriously. You need to be there for your kids in every way."

And with that the circle ends. The stick is passed around one last time so each student can break off a piece and take it home with them—a reminder, a touchstone to the promises, the hopes, the intentions that surfaced here. The Heartstick ceremony is nearly always a meaningful part of graduation. But on this day it was simply remarkable. Everyone, even younger brothers and sisters, was willing to play. No one was hiding out, no one afraid to try to tell their truth. Toward the end we were all looking at one another and smiling, like we knew without a word that we'd been beneficiaries of a strange and wonderful kind of communion, a level of kinship that most of us would have never believed possible. As for me, the whole three months was worth it just for this.

Diplomas are handed out, there are hugs and more tears still, promises to stay in touch. And then slowly, one by one, the families begin drifting back down the road, through the pines that line the creek to the parking lot. They get in their rented cars, take one last look at Boulder Mountain, drive off to whatever lives are waiting down that twisted highway.

EPILOGUE

WHEN AT THE age of twelve, the future Shawnee leader Tecumseh blackened his face with soot and bear grease and walked out of Chillicothe on the quest of his young life, to find his spirit helper, he was hungry, scared, and utterly alone. Not a single person in the village acknowledged him as he made for the Miami River and the high, wooded bluffs beyond; not a single hunter or foot traveler who passed him on the trail acted as if he even existed. More than the mosquitoes, more than the rain and cold that soaked and chilled him through the dark nights of fasting, it was that separation, that aloneness, that hurt most.

The same might be said of the kids who left their tribe in the burnt canyons and wooded uplands of southern Utah. One minute tethered to a community that traded every single day in the language of beauty, terror, dreams—the sacred mingling with the mundane—the next minute back in school, at the mall, on the street corner, with old friends or new, but almost certainly with no one who could understand.

Just as staff predicted would happen, the early months beyond the wilderness would bring many of the kids profound ordeals—drugs again, stealing, feelings of hopelessness; the real rites of passage, some call it. Like Tecumseh, in the worst of those times they would at least have a *pawawka* of sorts to lean on, a tenuous but valuable sense of choice, cobbled together out of something forged in the throes of their worst days in the wild. But unlike Tecumseh, who ended his quest by walking back into the arms of a culture that cherished his suffering, committed to helping him invest it with meaning, many of these kids have walked out of their ordeal into villages that plain don't give a damn. We so regularly portray the trials of our young people—drugs, violence, gangs—as the greatest of tragedies. But how much bigger a tragedy to watch them struggle through such experiences, inch their way clean of old ways, only to brush them aside, leave them to weave out of whole cloth a village of their own. A few good friends from rehab. Maybe a brother or a sister. If they're lucky, a mom and a dad.

The fact that this kind of experience is providing so many kids with their first chance for quiet, their first feeling of community, first glimpse of beauty, first sense of acceptance, says less about the abundance to be found in the last wild places than it does about the lack of it in the world beyond. "It can be difficult to fit what I learned out there into daily life," Susan tells me in a letter seven months after graduation. "I guess that's because we placed emphasis on such different things than modern society does—introspection, values, teamwork, and acceptance, instead of money, greed, and power."

The story of one student-turned-instructor, Ben, a twenty-two-year-old with a calm voice and deep-set eyes, is typical of how things often play out in the wake of the wilderness.

Ben says that when he got out of this program the money from his family's insurance was used up. Gone. No option of going on to some other program to try to anchor what he'd learned in the wild. He describes the shift out of the safe, positive community he'd helped build in the wilderness, back to the same old party friends in high school, as the most awful experience. "A few weeks after getting back I got high during a lunch break. It was a big high, because my body was so clean. I was supposed to take a VCR from the library up to a classroom and I freaked out—ended up going into a stall in the bathroom and crying for hours. My parents were so up on how well things were going for me since I'd gotten back from Utah, I just couldn't tell them. I couldn't do it."

Things went downhill from there, and it wasn't long before Ben's parents knew exactly what was going on. One day his father, who Ben says was never much of a disciplinarian, in what would be one of the most painful moves of his life, called a locksmith to change the locks on the doors, shutting his son out for good. "They basically said, 'Hey, we've done this thing for you, given you this experience, and you've pulled us in emotionally. Now you're back in the shithole and there's nothing we can do anymore.'"

One day Ben took Ecstasy and LSD, then went off to play basketball with some friends. During the game he dislocated his shoulder, and when they took him to the hospital he was given a shot of morphine. After that he took a bunch of Quaaludes. "I started hallucinating, and it went on for almost two weeks. When I finally came down I knew that was it, that was the bottom, and I had to get out. When I was out in the wilderness I'd made a real spiritual connection. The desert, the bow-drill fires, going on a quest. That's what made me know I couldn't allow myself to go any lower. If I hadn't had that powerful experience I wouldn't have known there was another way. It would have been so much harder. I knew I had to pick myself up out of the shit, and that's what I did. That's when I started leaning on what I learned in this program. I knew how to process stuff, how to approach problems, how to tell the truth. It was back to being a coyote all over again, having to figure out how to do reality checks, how to take care of myself. And it's ten times more difficult on the outside."

Ben says he thought seriously about going back into a rehab program, but in the end decided that what he really needed was another solo, another experience in the wilderness. Take as little as possible and just go. And that was the real start of a new beginning. He still does the same thing whenever life isn't going well, whenever he needs to think. "I know a lot of students who end up doing solos when they get out," he says. "They don't know what else to do. Most are reluctant to tell anybody they're struggling because their parents, all their friends, think they're fixed. Sometimes it just hurts too much to tell them otherwise."

Eventually Ben made his way not just out of the hole but back to the wild, back to his community, where he helps other kids going through the same kinds of struggles he faced. In truth, many of the kids I was in the program with who are now doing especially well seem inclined, just like Ben, to build some level of giving into their lives—volunteering, tutoring, planning careers in helping professions.

I begin reconnecting with kids about a month after walking away from that grad site on the flank of Boulder Mountain, along Grouse Creek, in the ponderosa pines. It's then that I get my first call from Susan, beside herself with excitement, eager to tell me about an honest-to-goodness ceremony she'd put together back home. During the program she'd missed becoming an eagle by inches, mostly because she ran out of time before she could complete a couple of small items necessary for the transition. Still, she'd come so far, had done so incredibly well in those eight weeks, at her good-bye group a couple of the staff quietly handed her an eagle bead, told her she'd know when the time was right to place it on her necklace and make it hers. That time, she told me, had finally come.

It happened at her grandmother's house. "It was so important to me that she be there," she said. "And her second husband, who died last winter—he'd been like a grandfather to me. I wanted to feel like his spirit was with me during this." Susan started by setting up a circle of five chairs out in the yard—for Grandma, for Mom and Dad, for her sister and brother. In the center of the circle she laid a towel, on the towel a candle, and next to that, an arrowhead and four special stones she'd carried with her for weeks down in Utah. Everyone took their seats; she walked alone down the long driveway through the woods, then back again. "I did that to clear my head," she explained. "To have a chance to reflect on what I was about to do."

She entered the circle and sat down in the center, and one by one, each family member read a poem or passage she'd given them that held special meaning for her. Afterward her sister tied that piece of sinew around her neck, the one Jenna had laid in her palm at Yarrow Springs three months earlier, the necklace that was "empty to remind you the time has come to begin adding new things to your life." Now it had three beads on it: one for coyote, one for buffalo, one for eagle.

For many kids the ordeal, the rite of passage that comes later, back in this world, has to do with drugs or booze. Not so for Susan. In a sense hers has been an even harder passage, a wrestling match with a monkey that will likely never completely give up on her, a depression that may be stitched into the fabric of her life for all the days to come. The crisis happens in late fall, when she overdoses on medication again, seriously, enters the hospital not through the suicide ward but through intensive care. The men and women who've been mixing the pills can't seem to find a formula that will bring her relief. In the end they opt for electroshock therapy.

A few weeks later I pick up an e-mail from her. She says she's found a piece of wood and can't figure out what it is— she thinks it may have to do with the wilderness program, but isn't sure. Wonders if I have any idea. I do. It's the piece of the Heartstick she broke off at the end of graduation back in June, on that warm summer day in Utah when the air smelled like burning sage and we all looked at one another across that circle and knew it was one of the finest moments in our lives. When I hang up the phone I'm so damn depressed I could cry.

———

Soon after that bit of heartbreak I climb in the van and head south again, back to Utah, this time to visit with Ray, Sara, and Beth, all of whom are in aftercare at a resident program just outside Loa. The four of us amble back and forth along a dirt road that cuts along the edge of a sprawling field of cheatgrass and sage.

"This is an all-right place," Ray tells me. "Some of the staff are great. But when I got here there were forty kids, and now there are sixty. They can't keep track of it all. They don't have the time for us like they used to."

Ray is just three months away from turning eighteen, at which point he can sign himself out of here and never look back. He says he's thinking of going on to college, though he hasn't decided in what. It's a bit of a shock to hear him even talking about such a move, considering what his view of school in general was when I met him. The first day we sat together out in the desert south of Trapper Ridge, he read me a poem he'd written called "Public School," a sour portrait of his so-called education: learning how to make bongs out of beakers and test tubes in science class; in math, how to divide drugs up for his friends:

> My English teacher's a lazy fuck
> who doesn't like to read.
> He taught us words like tits and ass
> Things we really need.
>
> In history we learned about the 80s,
> Bad music and cokeheads.
> We learned about these great explorers,
> Their names were Bill and Ted.

Two months after he got out of the wilderness Ray and a
couple of other kids bolted from the boarding school back into
the woods of Boulder Mountain—a move he says had a little to
do with being anxious, restless, and a lot with missing the freedom of the field. "For a little while it was great. I mean we were
all kids from the wilderness program, so we knew how to survive up there. Then one night we headed down into Bicknell,
stole this truck, were heading for Las Vegas when a cop stopped
us for not having any taillights. He knew who we were right
off."

It's the telling of the tale that's different now. Six months
ago Ray would have spun this out as a consummate war story,
working in all sorts of bravado. Now there's no pride in it at all.
He responds to my questions about the incident but offers not
a shred of color. "I've been good ever since," he says several
times. "I've even made Discovery," referring to a fairly high
level of leadership here at the school. It's like the drugs and the
running are part of what Ray thinks of as the behavior of a boy,
and right now he's reaching hard to be a man. Even that great
dream of one day heading off to Mexico with Frank to meet
Castaneda's Yaqui Indians seems to be running out of steam, in
favor of the attempt at college.

At one point the four of us sit on the ground, and the kids
ask me for a story—something I used to tell in the field—so I
offer the Ojibwa tale, the one about how butterflies taught children to walk. Afterward they're quiet, looking out to the north
across the sweeps of sage. "I miss the field so much," Beth
finally says, a comment seconded by Ray and Sara without a
breath.

"But you all hated it at first," I say, wondering if to some extent they might be engaging in that favorite hobby we all share in, editing the past. "By four or five weeks into it none of us hated it," Sara informs me matter-of-factly. "There was structure and all that, but we were free. Being out there in that setting, in all that nature, we never felt closed in. We never felt cornered."

"Besides," Beth jumps in, flashing a whimsical look, "out there I had this feeling of being able to take care of myself. I knew how to get warm, stay dry, build a fire. It was like I had some personal power, and it happened every day, over and over again."

It was the first program ever, they all agree, that they couldn't bullshit their way through. "There was no place to hide," explains Beth. "Sooner or later you had to work on your stuff. That's one of the things that scares me about going home; back there it's so easy to just disappear."

I tell her that's interesting to hear, because a lot of people would say running off to the wilderness is a kind of hiding out from your problems. She gives a little snort, shakes her head. "Yeah, right."

"Say you go into a psych ward," Sara tells me, and Sara is definitely no stranger to psych wards. "It's no big deal if you do anything or not. If you want to lay around, you lay around. If you want to watch television, you watch television. It doesn't matter. That wasn't true in the wilderness. Out there what you did mattered a lot." She sounds curiously like noted psychiatrist Thomas Lowry. Thirty years ago he talked with great urgency about the fact that while institutions may have the best of intentions, by taking care of a patient's every need, by making what they do more or less irrelevant, they've created a situation "where the patient's original feeling of worthlessness is confirmed." The farther in both time and distance the patients get from the hospital, said Lowry, the saner they become.

But, then, Sara could have told you that.

As for some of the rest of the tribe, Kevin is at a resident boarding school doing better than even he expected. "I've stayed clean," he says in a letter. "I'm getting stronger." Nancy, on the other hand, went on to an eating disorder clinic in Colorado for two months, in an effort to try to get a better grip on her bulimia. There were good people there, her mother tells me shortly after she leaves that program for a resident boarding school. "I'm sure she learned things she'll use in the years to come. But she was used to being outdoors, being free. She loved that so much, and at the clinic she was completely confined. She was hurting. I think it got in the way."

The saddest story by far in the early months is Keith's, the wiry kid I picked up with Kevin and Susan in Salt Lake City, the "possible runner" who became an eagle. Thrilled with their education consultant's recommendation of the program in southern Utah, Keith's parents turned to him again for suggestions on aftercare. He recommended a school in Virginia. His father says it was the worst experience of his son's life.

"Keith was so strong when he came out of Utah. For the first time in years he was really motivated to put new things into his life. We lost all that in aftercare." Rick says the program in which he ended up placing his son went way beyond discipline; in fact, he likens it to a concentration camp. "We went down to see him after a month, and I couldn't believe it.

Kids were routinely standing at attention before meals for an hour in one-hundred-degree heat. There were mosquitoes and flies all over them, and they couldn't swat them; we saw one kid who did, and he was severely disciplined. When we pulled Keith out he was sick, had red welts all over his body—the doctor said he was reacting to toxic levels of bug poisons. Four months later you could still see the red marks on him. Look, I have no problem at all with a strict program. But my son was brutalized."

With great sadness Rick tells how after that experience Keith completely lost interest in what anybody had to say to him. His focus went back to drugs, and drugs alone, and he did whatever he had to do to get them. Nine months later he would be crisscrossing the country, getting kicked out of one school and going into another, drifting, resentful, closed off. In late winter the therapist at the resident school Keith was attending said he had "about a zero chance" of going back out on the street and not becoming a junkie.

By the time spring rolls around, close to a year after the kids first went into the wilds, most are doing pretty well. Kevin, from Group 4, has been off drugs for six months now. Jenna washed her hands of the twenty-six-year-old guy who used to beat her; she's also staying physically strong, running five miles every day. Brenda is back at home—still having trouble with her mother, still acting out now and then, but enjoying great success in school. She says she wants to go to an Ivy League college, and what Brenda wants, something tells me, Brenda will get. Larry, the kid who lay down in a sleet storm trying to kill himself, is still soaring like an eagle; he's finishing up at boarding school, got accepted into Purdue University, plans to study engineering.

After some rough sailing, continuing her dance with bulimia, Nancy is doing better, is at least engaged in her classes. She turns eighteen in two months, old enough to blow off the boarding school, but has decided to stay—says it's the best place for her right now. In late spring I talk with her mom and dad, and while they sound a bit weary from all the drama of the past year, there's still some measure of hope in their voices. They say they know full well now that the bulimia could kill her, that if she keeps going there could be severe damage to her internal organs. They sound resigned, as all parents must finally be, to the fact that they cannot tell her a new way of thinking, instruct her on what matters in life— they can give support, but whatever change happens will have to come from her.

"To this day," her father tells me, "Nancy is more proud of having made it through that wilderness program than anything else in her life." He says it left her confident she could pretty much do whatever she wanted, at least when the bulimia is under control. "It was just one part of the journey. But it was an important part."

At the end of our conversation I ask her father if he would do anything different bringing up his daughter, if knowing what he knows now, he would change his approach to parenting. "Yes," he says. "I would've worked a lot harder to instill in Nancy a sense of what's really important in life. I'd've put a lot more effort into countering the terrible effects of advertising, all the things the culture tells us are valuable—looks, status—things that have nothing to do with the real value of life at all."

I have to tell you, Susan continues to surprise me. In April she calls to talk about the latest frustration with her medication, how the doctors have her on a sleeping agent mixed with Prozac and it takes her five hours to even wake up in the morning. On the other hand she's just passed her GED ("no sweat"), has been accepted at Indiana University, where she plans to study psychology, and is trying her best to get into the Peace Corps. "When I was down in Utah I found out I could do all sorts of stuff I never would have thought possible. I was responsible for myself, every day. It left me not afraid anymore to try new things." In her weekly support group Susan says she often talks about her time in the wild. "It helps me keep 'the fire within,' " she explains, referring to an image from the Tecumseh story she read on her first solo, where every day the young boy Tecumseh had to keep going back to that cold river and jumping in.

It's when I tell her it sounds like she's not letting the depression slow her down much that she says the most amazing thing of all: For the first time ever, she's come to see her illness as a kind of gift, something that leaves her deeply thankful for the good things, the good days in her life. "It started last November, after the whole intensive care thing. I came out of that and, I don't know, life just seemed more precious. There's so much to be grateful for. I don't think most people have that kind of perspective."

Developmental psychologist Juan Pascual-Leone, talking about the challenges that face people in later life, said that the key to forging what's commonly called wisdom lies in learning to cope with loss. He could just as easily have been talking about the kids in that wilderness program, so many of them with losses reaching far beyond their years: losses of innocence and identity, of friends to drugs and violence; losses of family, losses of hope. And yet, true to Pascual-Leone's point, those who make it through, and sometimes even those who don't, do now and then seem awfully wise.

The majority of native cultures have long believed that older people, the wise ones, are naturally linked not with their own children but with those who stand two generations away; it's the young, they say, who give honest voice to what is stirring in the culture at large. In America, it seems, are these same two groups, standing on opposite sides of life and leaning toward each other, separated by a society disconnected from both. One day soon, of course, you and I will be the old ones. Maybe then it will dawn on us that when it comes to the young, it was never about anything more than just being there, listening—that with nothing more than that we could have taught them that they mattered after all.

It was a long time ago, and the Great Spirit was in the middle of creating this very patch of desert—right where we're sitting—when suddenly he was called away. No one remembers exactly what was going on, but you could tell it was important because the Great Spirit wasted no time in leaving; reached into his pocket and tossed out the handful of junipers you see around you, these few pinches of grass, a couple of handfuls of flowers: that globe mallow and paintbrush over there. This pepperbrush. The evening primrose along the road. And then he was gone.

It was many years before he made it back, and when he got here, he was tired. The first thing he did was head over to the top of the Henry Mountains and just sit there, gaze out across this unfinished desert, try to figure out what to do with it. That's when he saw them. Far below, humans running around—men, women, children—not just living, but thriving in this roughshod place; squatting among the rocks, knapping arrowheads, twisting yucca into cordage, singing water out of the ground at Yarrow Springs. He was amazed that they could do so much with so little, and he found himself drawn to them because of it. Week after week, month after month, he sat up there and watched. And then one day he decided to come down and live in the midst of those nomads, those forgotten ones.

And it was a good time to be alive. The Great Spirit right here, resting in the heartbeat of the people's drums. Showing them how to dance, how to find their voice. Teaching them to hear their own breath in the whisper of a raven's wings.

AFTERWORD

People say that what we're all seeking is a meaning for life. I don't think that's what we're really seeking. I think that what we're seeking is an experience of being alive . . .

—Joseph Campbell

A warm spring day in Missoula, Montana. In the back of a restaurant on Spruce Street, I sit at a tall table listening to Sara. It's hard to believe this is the same young woman who a decade ago I knelt beside at a dry wash in the Red Desert, a rough scowl spilled across her face as she hurled curses at Jonathon, at the therapists, at her parents. Locked up tight, letting no one in. Today she seems enthused, accessible – grounded in the way of people who've had to fight hard for their wisdom, who understand that living well in the world takes a rather sophisticated set of skills. She tells me eagerly about having just finished her undergraduate degree in social work at the University of Montana - how next semester she'll be going on for her masters. "It wasn't all great after I got out [of Aspen]," she suddenly offers, breaking from her current life to recount some tough times in a boarding school. "The therapy at a place can be okay or not. But without some level of nature as part of the experience, it's just not going to be as powerful."

While most of the kids I followed went on to lead fairly urban lives, it would be ongoing considerations of nature that drove many of our conversations, some ten years after they walked off the stony plateaus of southern Utah. Susan continued to return to the canyon country for visits, seeking the feelings that for her came more easily there than anywhere on earth. Jenna and Nancy, on the other hand, never returned, though for many years they've had firm habits of taking regular walks in whatever park or green space happens to be near. "Aspen worked for a lot of us," says Jenna, "first because it connected us with nature. But also because it connected us for such a long time. No matter what conversations you might be having in therapy, you can usually find a connection with nature. It was enough to change my perspective about who I am. About what it means to be human."

Out in the wilds with their group, I was told – echoing sentiments expressed back in 1998 - for the first time in their lives these young people had been part of something bigger than themselves. On one hand that was expressed every day in essential fashion – carrying group supplies up the trail, cooking meals together, talking to the new kid who can't get a handle on his fear. "Most teens don't feel all that relevant," Larry told me recently. "We say we crave freedom. But that freedom is at its best when it gets connected to something that counts." In later years, this sense of connectedness would play out in a variety of ways. Out of the nine kids I got in touch with again, seven had at one time or another pursued some path meant to "give something back." Several entered so-called helping professions, be it nursing, social work, or psychology; others had done or were still doing volunteer work – literacy programs, math tutoring, even drug counseling. "I went to Aspen thinking how bad off I was," said Larry. "I was obsessed with all the wrongs I'd suffered." By the time he left the program, he says the world was bigger. It was no longer all about him being a victim.

Others put it in more basic terms. "Sometimes I wonder," says Carla, "how much of my success was just simplifying the world to the point where I could think straight. Maybe have a real conversation, watch a sunset, figure out what was going on in my head. Once you know what all that's worth, it's easier to commit to putting them in your life." Her comment mirrors well what seminal environmental researchers Rachel and Stephen Kaplan have been saying for thirty years. Nature, they explain, offers critical time away from everyday problems. That opening, combined with what the Kaplans call "soft fascination" - large movements and processes, from weather patterns to river flows, which while intriguing don't require focused attention – provides a powerful opportunity for restoration.

When I asked the students recently if there was anything they'd change about their experience, a common response was that programs should work harder to provide ties to people who knew what they'd gone through. "It was so hard to talk about what happened out there," said Jenna. "Back home, nobody ever had that kind of experience." She says it would've been helpful if therapists there had been at least slightly familiar with what goes on in the field - if they could at least speak the language. "There was a time, maybe four or five months after I got back, when I started to wonder if some of the insight I'd gained about myself was all in my head. Like a daydream. It took me falling off the wagon to finally get it - to accept what I'd learned as really true." Having someone in your life who knew about wilderness therapy would be like having a witness. "It'd be harder to doubt what happened."

         *   *   *   *

Out of millions of teens who need professional help each year dealing with issues or addictions, probably less than twenty-five percent are getting it. For starters, our managed care system has left relatively few patient beds available for kids in trauma; as a result they either end up in hospitals, biding their time until appropriate services become available, or in many cases, enter a criminal justice system where reliable therapeutic intervention is harder to come by. Indeed, fully seventy percent of kids in the correctional system have been diagnosed with mental health issues; sixty percent are struggling with addictions. As noted researcher Dr. Keith Russell points out, the continuum of care so often talked about by behavioral healthcare experts – services in schools, outpatient, inpatient, day treatment, and accessible residential facilities – "appears to be a myth for most adolescents and their families."

As I mentioned at the beginning of this book, good wilderness therapy programs, while just one therapeutic step among many, are showing extremely positive results treating many of the most acute problems of our times - from attention deficit disorder, to anger issues, to drug addiction. Yet sadly, while there are more wilderness therapy programs out there than a decade ago, the profession as a whole has yet to receive its due. Mental health providers – or more accurately, the managed care system that drives them – are inclined to push for treatments that fit easily into the existing institutional juggernaut. This means powerful experience-based treatments of all kinds, from equine therapy to wilderness programs, are routinely relegated to the back burner, left as options mostly for families who can pay for them out of their own pockets. (Sadly, when several states did elect to fund outdoor programs in the late 1990's, the money was almost without exception given to boot camps, which for most kids have little or no value.)

Stuck in this institutional miasma, it's little wonder that over the past decade behavioral drug prescriptions have skyrocketed. In the 2005 school year alone, America's children were given more than 25 million prescriptions for Ritalin. "Too many people are responding [to these problems] with a quick fix," says Dr. Donald Cohen of the Yale University Child Study Center. "As a nation we should be reserving medication only for those situations when it's proven to be an effective approach and where we can't approach it in other ways." Oxford researcher Susan Greenfield goes further

still, worrying that the convergence of our heavy reliance on pharmaceuticals, combined with the constant feel-good dazzle of our
technologies, is creating a world where pleasure - or at least the
absence of pain - is perceived as the be-all and end-all of life.

*   *   *   *

On that fine spring day in Missoula, sitting with Sara, what
struck me most about her was the extent to which she'd made
peace with her fears. True, the world still wasn't always a safe place,
but then she no longer needed it to be. She no longer devoted a
lot of her energy simply to protecting herself. In the end – for her,
and for countless others – perhaps the greatest, most lasting value
of wilderness therapy was the gift of courage: Courage to be fully
present in your life. Courage to lay claim to your authentic joy, but
also, and just as important, to find a place for your authentic pain.

Among the most powerful messages that were delivered in
the wild – not by therapists or field staff, but by nature itself – was
that in the end there was simply nowhere to hide. Early on kids
ended up surrendering to the unexpected – be it the challenge of
a sudden rainstorm, or the delight of a magnificent sunset. In time
there came a feeling of being aligned with larger movements - the
ebb and flow of day and night, a clearing sky, the unfurling of a
season. And from that place, for reasons we may never understand,
there arose in many a clear sense of what needed to be done. The
feeling of life as an arrow finally free of the archer's hand – in flight
at last and away, moving surely, unavoidably toward the heart of
what we may be.

Gary Ferguson
April, 2009